Feedback from part....

Dancing With Fear is a wonderful book of stories, told in many voices, about the experience of living with breast cancer. The reader may laugh or cry, agree or disagree with the numerous "healthful" hints. But one thing is certain; it is a healing labor of love for the author, the contributors, and all women, men, and children who have been touched by this disease.
    —*Shelagh Coinner, Psychotherapist, Nurse, breast cancer survivor*

Writing about my experience with breast cancer has felt good. It's like digging in warm soil in the spring with my hands.
    —*Sheryl, breast cancer survivor*

I thoroughly enjoyed reading the book—it was interesting and enlightening to see the range of experiences and our responses to them. I could relate to most of the people and for those I couldn't relate to, I marveled at our differences. This book offers practical tips to survivors and friends, and I found the read therapeutic even 13 years after my initial diagnosis!
    —*Donna Tremblay, breast cancer survivor*

Live for today, smile a lot and remember. . . when the sun comes up, you can do anything. We all have choices and decisions to make so make them wisely, and enjoy every moment you have. Life is wonderful.
    —*Gwyn Ramsey, breast cancer survivor*

When you go through cancer, isolation can be all encompassing. Often your support system needs you to be a stoic hero so that they can support you. Leila's *Dancing With Fear* realistically provides the reader who does not have cancer compelling stories of the depth of emotion cancer patients experience and how those supporting them can be of comfort. For the warriors of cancer, the stories provide important advice and illuminate the hopes, dreams and fears that make all survivors kindred spirits.
    —*Heather Resnick, breast cancer survivor*

Thank you for letting me tell my story. I found it to be a very cathartic experience. I hope others will find hope and strength in the pages of your book.   —*Rita, Santa Clarita, CA, breast cancer survivor*

Thanks for doing this book to help others with breast cancer. It was therapeutic for me just to write about this.
    —*Joni, breast cancer survivor*

Survival is triumph enough. (Harry Crews)

DANCING WITH FEAR

Tips and wisdom from breast cancer survivors

May the strength of three be in your journey. (Irish Proverb)

Leila Peltosaari
Tikka Books

Dancing With Fear:
Tips and wisdom from
breast cancer survivors

Tikka Books
P.O. Box 386, Verdun Post Office
Verdun, Quebec H4G 3G1 Canada

Photo: comstock.com
Layout: Albert Albala
Cover: RinaMaarit and Albert Albala
Copyright © 2005, Leila Peltosaari

www.tikkabooks.com
www.DancingWithFear.org

Library and Archives Canada Cataloguing in Publication

Peltosaari, Leila, 1947-
        Dancing with fear : tips and wisdom from breast
cancer survivors / Leila Peltosaari.

Includes bibliographical references and index.
ISBN-10: 1-896106-05-6
ISBN-13: 978-1-896106-05-2

        1. Breast--Cancer--Popular works. I. Title.

RC280.B8P44 2005   616.99'449   C2005-901777-5

Please visit www.tikkabooks.com and contact us for individual and quantity
orders. Quantity discounts are available for educational, business, and
promotional premium use, and for fund-raising. All rights reserved in all
languages. Printed in Canada.

To breast cancer survivors, past, present, and future.

Courage is not freedom from fear; it is being afraid and going on.
(Sir Philip Sidney)

Using This Book

While reading about the entire breast cancer journey is helpful and therapeutic, it can be frightening and overwhelming to anyone who is just starting out on this new road. Feel free to read this book either in its chronological order or by focusing on a specific chapter relevant to your situation. Whether you are reading for information, inspiration, courage or comfort, this book will guide you through it all, and you will realize you are not alone.

Contents

Using this book 5

Foreword 8

Dancing with fear 10

A life-changing moment 12
    Brief profiles of participants and events
    surrounding diagnosis

Dealing with the medical system 33
    Doctors, appointments, hospitals,
    what makes a good patient

Surgeries 46
    Lumpectomy, mastectomy, reconstruction,
    regaining arm movement

Lymphedema 69
    Dealing with it, avoiding it

Chemotherapy 76
    Coping with side effects, hair loss, favorite foods

Radiation 92
    Dealing with side effects, recovery

Tamoxifen and aromatase inhibitors 99
    Hormonal therapy drugs, dealing with side effects

Complementary and alternative treatments 107
    What might help, what might harm

Fear of recurrence 116
    Getting through fear, facing a new battle

Optimism and pessimism 127
　　　　What helps you to cope
Aftermath 136
　　　　Looking back when treatments are over
　　　　and cancer moves behind you
Support 149
　　　　What helps emotionally, physically, practically,
　　　　and best gifts, best and worst things to say
Reclaiming life 171
　　　　Going on with life, moving away from illness
Spirituality 185
　　　　Reasons for gratefulness, comfort from prayers
Facing death 190
　　　　Regardless of prognosis, facing the
　　　　possibility of dying
Humor 198
　　　　Laughter, the proverbial best medicine
Afterthoughts 207
　　　　More insight from survivors
Glossary 214
Bibliography 216
　　　　Web sites and books for surfing and reading
Acknowledgments 220
Index 222

Foreword

Although there are hundreds, perhaps thousands, of books about breast cancer, this one is like no other. If you have been diagnosed with breast cancer, you will feel comforted by the first-person stories told by women who share your diagnosis. If a loved one is undergoing breast cancer treatment, you will better understand what she is going through. The women in this book (and a couple of husbands) reside in Canada, the United States, and Europe. The youngest are in their twenties. All of them articulately share their experiences, fears, and hopes. Many books have been written by and for breast cancer survivors. The strength of this book is that women speak from their hearts to the hearts and minds of their readers. A bond is forged through shared experiences. Although we do not meet, we are in the same sisterhood.

One great benefit of this book is validation. Learning that other women have similar concerns—worrying about treatment decisions, enduring side effects, losing time from work, potentially passing on the disease to daughters, engaging in sexual relationships, fearing recurrence—is validating and normalizing. Normalizing these concerns offers comfort when you may feel profoundly isolated. Did you lose a best friend due to your breast cancer diagnosis? Are you having sexual difficulties as the result of treatment? Do you feel the stress emotionally of supporting everyone else? Do you grieve for the body you used to have? Do you worry that the cancer is metastasizing? If so, you are not alone and these concerns are normal.

Emerging on the other side of the cancer experience, many women feel their lives are changed for the better. Their priorities are in order. They learn to say no. They maintain a proper diet and exercise. They more often say "I love you." They value birthdays. They seize opportunities. They take time for themselves. They don't "sweat the small stuff," but do "stop to smell the roses."

When I was diagnosed with breast cancer twenty years ago, there were no national organizations offering support groups, no breast cancer awareness runs or walks, no large-scale fund raising for research, no advocacy groups lobbying in Washington, and no Internet for information. I gained knowledge by talking with women who had had breast cancer and combing the library for books and articles. How I would have loved this book back in 1985!

Leila Peltosaari and I have never met in person, but hope to one day soon. We have met by phone and email. A chance conversation on a business call led to our hearing about each other. Soon after, Leila called me on the phone. That was two years ago. Since then, Leila gathered all the information for this beautiful book. We are the beneficiaries. Keep it by your bedside and whenever you need comfort, validation, a boost in self-esteem, or emotional support, open it and you will hear the voices of friends who share your experiences.

I have learned many lessons during my twenty years as a three-time breast cancer survivor. I learned to become well informed. I learned to be an active participant in my treatment decisions. I learned that each woman reacts differently to the diagnosis. I learned that grieving for my pre-cancer life and body was normal. I learned that I needed to take time for myself every day. I learned to ask lots of questions of my doctors to avoid unwanted surprises. I learned that the Internet can be a valuable resource. I learned to be vigilant about my health. I learned that my body communicates with me and I must pay attention. I learned that I am in charge of my own health. I learned that the medical team works for me, that I hired them. I learned to say, "Why not me?" and not just "Why me?" I learned that breasts do not make me feminine.

Your breast cancer journey is uniquely yours, but you may find help and hope while getting to know the many women in this book. One more thing I learned is that other women with breast cancer are the ones who really understand. And that is what I value most about this book.

Bev Parker
Research Analyst
Y-ME National Breast Cancer Organization
Chicago, Illinois, USA
June 1, 2005

Dancing With Fear

"It's very serious," said the doctor on the phone, not wasting words, "you have cancer." My innocent security vanished. I was 53 and the summer of 2000 was already in August. One year after a clean mammogram, I had a lemon-sized, aggressive tumor invading my life and my family. We had to learn too much too fast and make life-altering decisions about treatments. All I could think of was this acute crisis at hand.

Time-consuming and exhausting both emotionally and physically, cancer became a priority to the exclusion of everything else. Appointments with many doctors, tests, and treatments filled my calendar for months ahead. It seemed too distant to imagine or trust that ordinary life would ever be mine again. Not an overnight killer if a killer at all, cancer allowed me time—time to get terrified and to learn about this disease, time to face regrets of the past and worries for the future. Then it was time for options and solutions, time to feel hope and to experience humor and contemplate life beyond treatments. I was just one of many; hundreds of women are diagnosed every day in North America alone with this alarmingly common cancer.

The sun kept rising every morning. Life went on with hidden benefits. The simplest things like a gust of wind or a simple ray of sunshine on my face were unexpectedly euphoric, as if I had never truly noticed them and as if I might never feel them again. An emotional break from a busy life rearranged my priorities so that I could see what really matters and could delete unnecessary details. Facing potential death was both sad and interestingly natural, even acceptable. Truly appreciating my normal life, now at peril, became profoundly rewarding.

I wanted to know others with breast cancer. Their survival became my lifeline of hope. This is a book I would have wanted to have when newly diagnosed with breast cancer. An easy read about a difficult subject, it is a visit from survivors in the comfort of your home, at your convenience. Responding to my invitation to participate in this book, one hundred and twenty-five women—as well as two men who had lost their wives to breast cancer—generously shared their experience with heartfelt replies to my many questions. They range through many ages, from women just getting married and starting a family to middle-aged women getting ready for retirement, and to others in their golden age, all celebrating good years and even decades of survival. A few are still in treatments and some have faced recurrence.

Through shared real-life experiences, the participants make this book a compilation of user-friendly tips and brief personal quotes to give insight, hope and help to those just starting on this challenging road. The tips have been combined and categorized for ease of use, with selected comments edited for brevity. In order to protect privacy and guarantee confidentiality, participants were offered a choice to remain anonymous or use a full name, just a first name, pseudonym, or initials.

In my early childhood, the word cancer signaled a frightful disease. Fifty years later, it still does. When cancer visited me, I changed emotionally while physical scars healed. Normal life now goes on with joy, appreciation, and ordinary frustrations, but this experience has made me vulnerable. I now know it can happen to me. I can never unhear the diagnosis of cancer. This is difficult to explain, but other survivors understand. Many participants commented on the title for this book and said that it describes exactly how they felt and still feel.

Each chapter first outlines briefly my own cancer journey. I structured this book into sections to follow the journey we cancer patients go through. You can open the book at any page and read as much or as little as you like, or focus on the chapter relevant to your own journey or of interest at that moment.

Many said they could never repay the help given to them to get through their cancer and that the best thing they can do now is to help others. That is the reason for this book. With hundreds of glimpses through a common journey, this book is the voice of many. Everyone is different, and everyone's story is unique. There are no right or wrong answers, since every feeling and experience is valid and valuable.

Acknowledging with honesty the sorrow and pain of breast cancer, this book also voices the women's irrepressible joy of life, courage, and humor with practical tips and wisdom to share.

Surviving together and helping others,
Leila Peltosaari

A Life-Changing Moment

Brief profiles of participants and events surrounding diagnosis

---

Enjoy what you can, endure what you must. (Goethe)

I was stunned with despair, unable to think coherently. Just a year after a clean mammogram, I had a Stage III invasive carcinoma of 6 cm, mixed ductal and lobular. I found it accidentally and unexpectedly. One ordinary summer day, I was standing with arms across my chest when my subconscious signaled that one breast was soft and one was hard. It was not even a lump but rather the entire breast surface that was hard. I ignored it for a week but my intuition kept nagging me, so I went to get the tests done. When the phone rang and the doctor gave me the verdict, my daughter was still sleeping. It was supposed to be such a happy day, planning her 20th birthday party.

My husband noticed something different in my right breast. I had no symptoms and nothing was found in my mammogram. The tumor was detected by ultrasound and confirmed by biopsy.
(Katariina Rautalahti, Järvenpää, Finland, first diagnosed in 1999 at age 41, recurrence in 2003 at age 45)

A very active mother, grandmother, gardener, traveler, painter. I had retired from my government job as a secretary just two years before. No warning signs. We were preparing to leave for the winter in our recreational vehicle for Mexico. The diagnostic screening tech phoned me and told me I had cancer. I nearly collapsed.
(Carole, Victoria, BC, diagnosed at age 57)

I visited my sister overseas when she was going through breast cancer before I knew I would be diagnosed, too. I saw her without hair, met her doctors, saw her taking the chemo, met other patients and listened to their stories. They all seemed to be calm with a sense of humor. It helped me to meet my own cancer. A routine checkup detected a lump in my right breast, but a mammo found a tiny tumor in left breast. I was very lucky, but my first reaction was disbelief. Me? Even me? No, no, not now, the timing is not right, I wish to postpone this to a later date, perhaps to age 90 with one foot already in the grave...

(Maarit)

I found a lump and some dense areas when I did a monthly self-exam. I was also pregnant so I thought the changes were due to the pregnancy. When I had a miscarriage, I waited two weeks for my hormones to settle down and see what was going to happen to my breast. It was extremely painful, and I could not even sleep on that side. The lump and dense area did not go away. The ultrasound and mammogram did not show anything requiring immediate attention. They told me to come back in six months. The needle biopsy had something different to say.

(Melinda Flynn)

Routine mammogram in 1996. I was reading a novel as I relaxed on my deck. My husband was busy packing all afternoon, because we were leaving for Nova Scotia early Monday morning and wanted to attend the Montreal Jazz Festival over the weekend. Then my gynecologist

It might not be as bad as it looks. Get informed about your options. This is your life.

Get involved with your treatments. Read and be an advocate for yourself. Learn the vocabulary of your illness so you are prepared.

Seek support and help from family and friends. Reach out to other cancer patients in the hospital waiting rooms. Talk about your situation.

Don't compare yourself to others. Every case is different.

Put yourself first and take care of your needs mentally and physically. Learn to say no.

Take time to rest. You will need all your physical and mental energy and courage.

Cancer hotlines are there for you for comfort and good information.

---

called... I wrote down the appointments and, at the end, wanted to finish my book. Reading has always been my anchor in times of crisis, and this was no different. Now the sun did not shine with the same glow, the garden was no longer green, and the book no longer held me with the same spellbinding intensity. My healthy energetic body had broken down. Immediately I saw the wall closing in around me. How much time was left for me? Could one phone call snatch everything from me? I knew intrinsically that my world had changed forever. I thought about the grandchildren that I would never hold, the wedding plans that I would never make for my younger daughter. I decided with my husband to wait until we were sure what the prognosis was to tell our children, relatives and friends. Time is too slow for those who mourn. I took comfort in repeating frequently, "Medicine is not a precise science." After the doctor confirmed my fears, I felt free to release all my pent-up tears. I wept uncontrollably. This was raw reality and I did not expect a soft landing. Illness is the doctor to whom we pay most heed. To kindness, to knowledge, we make promises only; pain we obey.

(Vivia Chow)

My late wife, Glenna, was a primary school teacher. I was widowed by the disease at the age of 33 and consider myself a breast cancer survivor. Glenna had likely been misdiagnosed. A later lumpectomy revealed a stage IV breast cancer. I don't often drink hard spirits. A friend came over with a bottle of scotch. I drank most of it, went outside into the snow and cried for many hours.

(Dr. Barry J. Barclay, St. Albert, AB)

Involved in community service. Chairman of local Board of Education. Highly stressful life, healthy low-fat, low-salt diet prepared at home with minimal processed foods. No warning signs obvious. I had been taking estrogen for ten years following a hysterectomy. No pregnancies. Mammogram showed microcalcifications.

(Anonymous, diagnosed at age 55)

I am 56 and a workaholic with no children. My breast cancer was diagnosed in 1996. It would not have been found if not for a mammogram. It was Stage I, a good thing, if there is anything good about cancer. I thought to myself, "Okay, here we go again." I have had two other bouts with cancer starting with melanoma when I was only 22 years old, then cervical cancer in 1980 at age 33. I think there is something wrong with my immune system, because obviously I am prone to cancer.

(Joy McCarthy-Sessing)

I was a very active and hard-working woman with a healthy diet. I was told my diagnosis by a surgeon as he sat with his back to me leafing through my chart.

(Shelagh Coinner, diagnosed in 1998 at age 56)

I am a lesbian physiotherapist/music teacher/hobby farmer, living in a remote area of central British Columbia. I was diagnosed in 2001 at age 52. It was found in a screening mammogram, which I had while taking lots of tests for debilitating fatigue.

(Judith Quinlan, diagnosed in 2001 at age 52)

I was sitting in a car waiting for someone when I felt a swoosh under my right armpit. Later that evening I felt a lump about a half inch in diameter. A surgeon biopsied it, but then my GP overlooked the words "suspicious cells." A mammogram and ultrasound showed nothing. I moved, went to another GP, because the lump was still there. He gave me antibiotics, but they didn't help. Finally he sent me to the hospital. Breast cancer was diagnosed 15 months after my first visit.

(Esther Matsubuchi, North Vancouver, B.C.)

I really had no warning signs except that I kept getting infections and just couldn't seem to stay well. I found a lump myself. I woke up from the lumpectomy crying and saying I didn't want to have cancer, so I believe I heard them talking while I was under. I was completely shocked. There was a history of cancer in my family but not breast cancer, and I never thought I would get it. It all seemed like a really bad nightmare.

(Lorraine Langdon-Hull)

I was experiencing sharp intermittent pains in my right breast. I was told during my checkup that it was hormonal and absolutely not breast cancer. My doctor recommended having a mammogram just to ease my mind. During a lumpectomy, my surgeon found additional DCIS, which was still encapsulated. I had a mastectomy. My cancer was Her2Neu positive, which is considered faster-growing and more aggressive than estrogen-positive breast cancers. I thought I would have a little surgery and be done with it. How naive.

(Catherine, Pointe Claire, QC , diagnosed in 2001 one month before age 40)

I found a lump myself. A mammogram followed, then ultrasound and needle biopsy. On Christmas Eve I received the biopsy results, and they were not good.

(Debbie Giroux, Langley, B.C.)

It was a great shock to me, as I had no risk factors, no family history, and no symptoms. I worked out regularly, rode my bike everywhere, ate a low-fat, high-fiber diet, nursed both of my children till they were well over a year and had never taken the pill.

(Dawn, Victoria, BC)

Breast cancer runs in my family, so I was always aware of the disease. I found a lump in my left breast while doing a self-exam. With my age and my breasts being so dense, they could not see anything from the mammogram. After an ultrasound, a needle biopsy and a needle aspiration, I had a lumpectomy, and they removed the tumor and seventeen lymph nodes, all cancerous. I had another lumpectomy, as they didn't have clear margins from the first. The oncologist immediately sent me for more tests, including a bone marrow test, where it was discovered the cancer had spread to the bone marrow as well.

(Kathy Reeve, North Vancouver, B.C., diagnosed in 2000 at age 32 with metastatic breast cancer)

Writer, medical transcriptionist, diet on the healthy vegetarian organic side, took lots of supplements. Had Stage III ductal carcinoma with a 10 cm tumor. Found by self-exam. I knew when I found it that it was cancer. Massive relief upon diagnosis—"now I can get rid of it"— although my husband almost fainted. I saw image of many doors opening with light pouring through.

(Suzanna Stinnett)

I was a full-time college teacher who swam a mile twice a week and ate more than ten servings of fresh fruit and vegetables every day before I was diagnosed with inflammatory breast cancer. My warning sign was a red breast, but every time I went to one of the four doctors I saw in the four months before my diagnosis, it was not red. I also saw my skin go white as if it had no blood at all. The doctors kept saying, "But it doesn't look like cancer." Right, it didn't look like the cancers they had previously seen, but an oncologist or a breast surgeon, had I seen one, would have known. A punch biopsy performed by a dermatologist found the cancer. I believed what he was saying, but I couldn't take it in.

(Maria Hindmarch)

I can't believe it. I have no history, don't smoke, don't drink, I nursed all my babies, did everything right and here I am. At ER, they told me I had a breast infection, gave me antibiotics and sent me for a mammogram. A surgeon told me I have lumpy breasts and "nothing to worry about." Two years later my new doctor asks about my lumpy breast and wants a second opinion. After a mammogram, ultrasound, and a biopsy, I'm sitting in an oncologist's office and he's telling me I have cancer. I didn't want to know what stage, I couldn't handle it then. They put me on antidepressants, because I was a nervous wreck. My stomach had been in knots for three weeks, my whole world is turned upside down, and they wonder why I'm stressed.

(Linda Bryngelson, New Brighton, MN)

Over the years I had many, many cysts aspirated so lumps were nothing new to me. When I was 48, however, they called me back for a fine needle biopsy on two lumps, one in each breast. My gynecologist suggested I see a breast surgeon and thought I might as well get rid of this mass. This is where things started to go wrong. I went to the surgeon expressing concern about the lump in the left breast that was "solid." He looked at the mammogram and said they just didn't use a large enough needle and that he could collapse it. He then aspirated a number of cysts in my breast. This was a big mistake and an important lesson that I learned... always, always get a copy of the reports and let them speak for themselves. I didn't know until two years later that I had expressed concern for the wrong lump. The one in the right breast, from which fluid had been extracted, had the suspicious cells. Nothing had been done about this and I didn't go back for the 2-month follow-up thinking I had already dealt with the problem. When I was 50, I was diagnosed with invasive ductal carcinoma in that same area of my breast.

(Rita, Palos Verdes, CA)

I was a manager of a candy store at the time I found my lump at age 44 by doing my monthly breast self-exam. There were no warning signs. I really wasn't that upset, as my Father had passed away in 1978 from lung/brain cancer and my sister a few years later from colon cancer. So when I was diagnosed in 1990 it didn't really surprise me that much. I just felt it was going to happen sooner or later.

(Marianne Svihlik)

I was diagnosed in January 2000, just when I was thinking the millennium was going to bring great things my way. During the biopsy, they said, "Don't worry, probably only fibrocystic disease." I thought I led a healthy lifestyle, ate right, exercised, etc. My job is stressful, mostly because I take it on headfirst and, of course, "nobody can do it as good as me." First reaction? Can't be, there's none in my family, how come "she" doesn't have it... all the typical responses. But then it became, "Okay, why not me? And how am I going to get through this?"

(Rebecca Simnor)

Very busy lifestyle. I would exercise early in the morning several times a week. Diagnosed at age 32 with no warning signs. The lump was discovered by my gynecologist. After a mammogram, ultrasound and four stereotactic core needle biopsies, the radiologist told me one of the biopsy sites was cancerous. Fortunately, my brother, who is a physician as well, came with me to that appointment and that helped ease the enormous burden a little. I was completely dumbfounded and numb, was not expecting it at all. Not at my age, not now.

(Dikla, North Hollywood, CA)

My mom had breast cancer, twice. I've always been a little overweight, but as an adult I exercised vigorously. I had my first child later in life, at age 38. So I was just a walking set of risk factors. I had found a lump while breast-feeding my son when he was about 8 weeks old. The OB and I agreed to watch it, as it could have been a blocked milk duct. After I stopped nursing my son, the lump seemed to disappear, and then it reappeared about four months later. I had a mammogram, an ultrasound, and a core biopsy. The radiologist was sure it was benign. When he called me at work, I was not surprised but a little stunned and pretty numb. My first reaction was "shit... now I have to deal with this... this sucks." Not that I was worried about losing my life to cancer, I was more worried about losing my happiness to cancer.

(sams mom)

I detected my cancer in 1995 at age 54. I noticed puckering and dimpling on my breast as I stood in front of the bathroom mirror, putting my hair up after my shower. My mother had died of breast cancer and my father of colon cancer, and there were other cases of cancer on both sides of my family. My parents were raised in the Okanagan farming and orchard area of B.C. and had been subjected to the spray from DDT and pesticides while growing up. They were heavy smokers as well. I felt too busy to call the doctor and make an appointment and had put it out of my mind until I had a dream... I awoke in the middle of the night *knowing* that I had breast cancer. I believe that our mind, body, and spirit are all interconnected. After diagnosis, I was trying to be brave while hoping to make everyone else feel okay about my diagnosis. We women are so good at wearing a mask and protecting others at our own expense. I drove home and called a friend. I heard her crying, and her response seemed to act like a trigger. I began to weep softly for the first time since I found the thickening, and the thoughts of my mother and her battle with breast cancer came in the flood.

(Sharon Tilton Urdahl)

Receptionist, high-stress job. Obese, diagnosed at age 52 in 2000. No warning signs. Discovered by mammogram. No second opinion. I knew, I knew, I knew. I was able to take a trip with my daughter that long Labor Day weekend and go on with life even though my gut told me it was cancer. This was my fourth bout with "lumps."

(psh)

Here's the truth. I had to convince my doctor at age 35 that I needed a baseline mammogram (the first mammogram a woman has). I was an aerobics instructor at my ideal weight, fit, and had no family history of breast cancer. Five years later I marched in for an annual mammogram. Much later I found out that the doctors could diagnose me immediately from the mammogram, because I had that baseline mammogram at age 35. I had DCIS in the earliest of stages. I was extremely lucky and thank God that my father was a doctor, because without his guidance and intervention I would have been lost.

(Mary Schmidt)

I was diagnosed in 2000 at age 30. I had no family history or prominent risk factors. My daughter was 19 months old. I was utterly and completely shocked and blindsided. My doctors were all amazing, and I did not feel the need to seek a second opinion. The cancer was multifocal and large. I would fluctuate between thinking everything was going to be OK and that the scans were going to show cancer all over my body. Scans were clean. Happier words I'd never heard.

(Julie Austin, Little Rock, AR, diagnosed in 2000 at age 30)

I was diagnosed in 1985 at age 40 after finding a lump doing self-exam. My first reaction: I was like a marble that had just been smashed by a hammer. Each little piece was an emotional reaction, an avalanche coming all at once.

(Bev Parker, Naperville, IL, diagnosed in 1985 at age 40, recurrence in 2001)

I was a driven businesswoman at that time, a happy marriage, two wonderful children, a beautiful new home... the perfect picture of the successful American family. Breast cancer did not run in my family at all. I thought I was in great health. I was 37 when I discovered a lump in my breast about the size of a walnut. I was heading to the shower early one morning and instinctively reached to feel the lump. My gynecologist of 20 years told me it was nothing, even patted my shoulder to tell me that I was all right. Thirty days later I went back to him and asked him to check it again, and again sixty days later at which time he said why don't I have a mammogram. Days later I called back to ask the results and the nurse told me the results were fine. The results really said that further diagnostic testing was needed. A year later from the time I discovered the walnut-size lump, it had grown to the size of a lemon and I again went to the doctor's office and a needle biopsy was done. Both the doctor and his nurse were trembling and visibly upset as the needle biopsy was performed. They immediately scheduled me with a surgeon. I did not have any warning signs of any type.

(Beverly Vote, Lebanon, MO, diagnosed in 2000 at age 37)

I think I was probably at my highest stress level. I was told that my mammogram would really hurt because I had a big cyst, but my doctor said not to worry. It started to hurt two months later so my GP sent me to the hospital to have it drained. A needle biopsy was done as well as an ultrasound and now I was quietly frightened. My first reaction was "just let's get this out of my body." The mammogram showed nothing, even though I could feel the large lump. The diagnosis was a 10 cm infiltrating lobular carcinoma with micrometastases to 6 of 20 axillary lymph nodes and a Stage IV. The huge lesson I learned from this is to know your own body. For about a day I blamed my GP but then realized that I had to take responsibility. Never again would I delay if I thought something was wrong with my body.

(Joan Fox, Victoria, BC)

My lifestyle has ranged from being plump and inactive to eating healthy and being active. Feeling good. Thank God, I was careful about getting my mammograms on time because my mother, sister, and niece had all survived breast cancer. I went for my routine mammogram and more pictures were needed. After the fourth one, the doctor said it could be nothing—but it would have to be proven to him. Both tumors were malignant. My reaction was, "Slow and steady wins the race." I didn't ever have a big emotional reaction. My method of coping is to educate myself and to move forward, taking action. I chose mastectomy. I wanted to be as proactive as possible.

(Deborah, diagnosed in 2000 at age 46)

I felt a need to get a mammogram. I had one not quite a year before, but something was telling me. The doctor didn't see the need to give me one so soon, but I insisted. I felt no lump, but a mammogram showed a spot. I had a fine wire put in to help with the biopsy, and I was shocked that it was cancer, since there is no cancer in the family. The doctor told me that it would have taken a couple of years before I would have felt a lump at which time I would be dead. I felt very lucky that I had listened to my inner voice. I get really mad when I hear reports saying mammograms are a waste of time. A mammogram saved my life.

(Chris Lengert, Campbell River, BC., diagnosed in 1996 at age 52)

In 1986, I was forty-five years old, walking approximately 10 miles a week, and enjoying life. One evening I watched the television program, 20/20. It was about women who were most apt to get breast cancer. I listened to the category list of family history of cancer, first baby after 30, beginning period at age 10. There were about eight to ten items, and I fit every one. A cold chill danced down my spine. That evening when I went to bed, I did a self-exam, the first one in my life. To my surprise, I felt a small nodule. The next day I made an appointment with my doctor and had my first mammogram. The results were not good. My world hit bottom. That evening we told our children. Mark, our 8-year-old son hugged me and said, "You can do this, mom." What encouragement! This brave little boy had been diagnosed with leukemia in 1979 at the age of five, and he just went through three years of chemo. I decided if he could handle cancer, so could I.

(Gwyn Ramsey)

I discovered a lump by accident, had it for about 8 months, waiting for my annual checkup with gynecologist. He said it was nothing. Six months later, I demanded a mammogram, as the lump hadn't gone away and it was hard. Twenty years earlier I had a cyst removed, and I remember the doctor saying that the dangerous lumps were usually hard. When I learned the bad news, I cried and cried and cried but then got better. Once back at home, the tears would start again and again.

(Laura, Navarra, Spain, diagnosed in 1998 at age 41)

I was always afraid of getting cancer because my mother died of breast cancer when she was 59. At the end of 1999, I noticed that I had a lump, but I only noticed it because it was so painful. I thought it was another fibroadenoma, since I'd had one before. My gynecologist said it felt like normal tissue, but she'd send me for a mammogram "if I felt I needed one." Nothing showed up. That's when I insisted something was there, so they did an ultrasound and sure enough, there it was. So the journey began.

(Leslie, Springfield, VA)

Routine mammogram. I got a second opinion as the surgeon was convinced we had to do a total mastectomy, and I was convinced he just wanted to fatten his wallet and as much as told him so. We became friends after that. My reaction was disbelief, as I am never sick.

(Pat Eveleigh, Vernon, BC, diagnosed in 1995 at age 52)

Healthy diet, mostly chicken and fish, fresh fruits and vegetables, sugar substitutes & diet soda now and then, coffee... Diagnosed in 2000 at age 35. No warning signs, no family history, don't smoke, drink little alcohol. Discovered through self-examination. I had breast implants, so I couldn't find many general surgeons who wanted to perform a needle aspiration. Shocked, scared and devastated initially. After networking for a couple of days and researching, I realized how lucky I was to find it so early. I became strong and determined to beat the cancer and survive to live a long life.

(Stephanie, diagnosed in 2000 at age 35)

I worked full time, became very involved in civic and neighborhood matters, volunteered too much on projects that I cared deeply about. I was stretched entirely too thin and became physically and, often, spiritually exhausted. Then a series of events were emotionally devastating to me, and I felt like I had run into a wall. The one that was always such a cheerleader for everyone else could barely get out of bed to get through my day. A doctor diagnosed "depression." Two months later, while in the shower doing my BSE, I found a lump in my left breast. Intensive grieving and tears, fear, and research followed.

(Janel Dolan Jones, Fort Worth, Texas)

I have been a Clinical Nurse Specialist since 2000 and became the facilitator for a Breast Cancer Education and Support Group. As fate would have it, I became the group's newest member. I was scheduled to give my first official presentation to the group about the importance of continuing self-breast exams. The night before my talk, I did my own self-exam while in the shower and found a lump in my left breast. During the ultrasound, I knew it was bad. Tears streamed down my face. I felt a black hole in the pit of my stomach. I tried to tell myself that maybe it wasn't cancer. Maybe it was something else. I was 34 years old.

(Lori Kaneshige, Honolulu, HI, diagnosed at age 34)

I have always been in good shape. I work out and watch what I eat. In my 55 years, I have never been sick except for colds. Then I got the call to come back in for another mammogram. No lumps, but some calcifications. That call makes you very nervous. After the second mammogram, I had a stereoscopic biopsy, which again no one thought would be anything, but it was.

(S.R., Columbus, OH)

I was 51 when diagnosed, 10 years younger than mom was when she was diagnosed. Mammogram found it, probably because I upset the technician and she really slammed my breasts flat. I knew it was cancer when she came back to say that more films were needed. I was angry, not because it was I, but because so many of us still get it.

(Deb Haggerty, diagnosed at age 51)

At age 36, with a successful career in corporate marketing, breast cancer was the last thing on my mind. I'd just returned from a dream vacation to the south of France with my boyfriend when I found the lump. It took about four weeks for the usual round of tests of mammogram, ultrasound, and fine needle biopsy. All inconclusive but suspicious. I elected to have the lump removed and while on the operating table, I heard those words every woman dreads, "You have breast cancer." There is no breast cancer in my family. I got a second opinion from another team of doctors. Everyone was in agreement that I needed chemotherapy and radiation. My first reaction was shock and then fear. At the same time I had a firm belief that I was going to be OK. I don't know why. I just knew I was going to be a survivor.

(Lee Asbell)

I was 47 years old when diagnosed in 1989. I had no warning signs. I found the tumor by accident when I dropped a pencil while doing a crossword puzzle in bed, and as I reached down my other hand touched my breast, and I felt a lump. My doctor diagnosed it as cancer just by "feel." My first mammogram did not "see" the tumor but you could see it by eye. My first reaction was, "But how? I breast-fed my daughter!" My daughter was 10 years old and I thought that because I breast-fed I was immune.

(Sherry Gaffney, diagnosed in 1989 at age 47)

As a 58-year-old who nursed four daughters (twins included) I did not see this coming. No cancer in family. I'm a nurse working the night shift in home health and have always had a phobia about anesthesia. Decades ago I worked in an oncology ward when the radical mastectomy was the only treatment available. I had no warning signs. Even after the second mammogram discovered the lump I had difficulty palpating it. Ultrasound and a biopsy probe that sounded like a cap gun took bits of the tumor. Tears were streaming down the sides of my face as I lay there, my mind reeling from wearing wigs to lopsided bras to never seeing my grandchildren. Still I kept thinking the doctor would call and say it's all been a big mistake. I was going out to a play when the doctor who performed the biopsy called to say the results were positive, and when she put me on hold to look at the calendar I threw a potato clattering into the vertical blinds. I was furious, hated her. How dare she! My 21-year-old found me crying and said, "We don't have to go out, Mom." I said we are not sitting home all night crying. I put on a lace bra over the biopsy dressing, donned a low-cut dress, and we were out the door.

(Diane Dorman)

I found the lump myself. I had a biopsy using ultrasound after several mammograms that were suspicious. During the biopsy they discovered a second, very small tumor that was also biopsied. The surgeon, a woman who specializes in breast surgery, came in and very matter-of-factly said that the tumors were cancerous and needed to be removed right away. My son, who was 25 at the time, was with me. When she left to get something, my son came over to me and laid his head in my lap, and we just looked at each other. I'm single, and I knew my life was about to change substantially. I did not get a second opinion. I had booked a cruise for my son and I, my "cancer cruise." We went away and had a blast. When we came back, I was sick and had to postpone surgery till I got better.

(Rita, Santa Clarita, CA)

I had an abnormal baseline mammogram and then a biopsy. The oncology nurse told me the news over the telephone while I was at work. It was an awful way to get the news, but I am not sure there was a better way. My first reaction was complete fear. I immediately sent an email to a friend with whom I work, while I was on the phone with the nurse. My friend came to my office and sat with me, while I got the details, and then she helped me to get myself together to drive home and tell family and friends.

(Cindy, Cedarburg, WI, diagnosed at age 41)

Active lifestyle. I eat a fairly good diet, with some fast foods on a rare occasion but primarily I cook nutritious meals. I had been married eight months when first diagnosed at age 29 in 1984. A small lump in breast was growing from the size of a dime to the size of a quarter in two months. I found it by self-check. I opted for the total mastectomy of my left breast with immediate reconstruction. First reaction was very scared and baffled, a bit lost. But after consultation with the doctor and plastic surgeon and the large support from my new husband and family, I felt very positive about the procedure.

(Roberta R. Nordby, Redmond, WA, diagnosed in 1984 at age 29)

My lump was discovered on a routine gynecological exam. It was 1974, and I knew nothing about breast cancer. There were only one or two breast specialists at that time. I was referred to a protégé of the famous doctor that had developed the radical mastectomy. He aspirated the lump with negative results and set an appointment for a "biopsy." This would be a lumpectomy today. I made him promise that he would not take my breast if it was cancer, as they did in those days. I didn't want to wake up to a surprise. I wanted the decision to be mine.

(Gloria J. "Mimi" Winer, Point Pleasant, NJ)

My very first mammogram was in December 1997. A spot was detected and arrangements made, but by then we were with in the middle of the Montreal Ice Storm. I am a senior high school teacher which meant no classes for 3 weeks, no heat or electricity in the house, broken telephone wires—in other words, no life. My appointment at the hospital was postponed. It was a hellish time even without dealing with the thought of cancer.

(Susan, Brossard, QC)

Because of the family history I was diligent about having my breasts examined. By the grace of God, one evening, my hand went to my breast and there was a lump. The doctors all assured me it was "probably nothing."

(Dawn, North Hollywood, CA, diagnosed in 2001 at age 47)

I've been married to my college sweetheart for almost ten years, and we have three beautiful children. I was diagnosed in 2002 at age 32, just two days before my son's first birthday party. I originally went to the doctor with strep throat and, while I was there, I had her check a breast lump I had found the week before. Everyone, considering my age, said it was most likely a fibroadenoma, a benign condition that usually affects women in their 20s, but the only way to be sure was to biopsy the lump. My lump was not visible in the mammogram but was evident on the ultrasound. Then I got the call that changed the course of my life. The hardest part of the diagnosis for me was telling my parents. My mom had lost her sister to breast cancer, so I knew hearing I had it would be very difficult. The next six weeks were crazy; in fact I don't have clear memories of much of it.

(Amy Murphy, diagnosed in 2002 at age 32)

I was a very mature student at a university, a wife and mother of two special-needs children. I found a lump while singing in the shower. I got answers after two weeks. I think doctors sat around a table and determined two weeks would be long enough to drive the patient mentally insane with anxiety and fear.

(Heather Resnick, Thornhill, ON, diagnosed in 1997 at age 43, recurrence in 1999)

I exercised regularly and ate fairly healthy. I am a health information manager in a long-term care facility. I found a hard lump in my left breast. The mammogram was negative and the sonogram was inconclusive. The biopsy showed my breast was full of cancer. I was alone in the outpatient surgicenter when the surgeon told me I had cancer. My friends wanted to stay with me during the procedure but I foolishly said no, because I didn't want them to take time off work. I was numb, in shock, and I just stared out the window until my husband came to take me home. There was no need to get a second opinion.

(Sheryl)

I took care of myself, ate a good diet and stayed active. I was diagnosed at the age of 35 but I had found the lump at 30. The lump was painful, but I was told it was probably a cyst and it would go away on it's own. It did not grow, and I did not worry. I started working out at a gym and the lump seemed to have grown overnight to the size of a half-dollar. I figured either I had strained a muscle or had an infection. Cancer never crossed my mind. I was not concerned, since breast cancer is not supposed to be painful (big myth). During my first mammogram I am waiting for the technician to tell me I may go to have my ultrasound done, and I overhear the doctor say, "That's cancer and I want you to do some more pictures." I think, "Wow, that poor woman!"—but they were talking about me. I am stunned and in shock. How can I have cancer? I am not old enough, it hurts, it's just a cyst, you are making a mistake! I am terrified. I am not thinking clearly at all. I just want to hear my husband's voice and to feel his arms around me to tell me it's all going to be okay. We cry, we curse, and we decide to kick the cancer's ass and win!

(Michelle Woods)

I was 52 years old and in excellent health. Our diet was and is wholesome foods, mostly made or cooked from scratch. My cancer was detected by annual mammogram. No lump, just a slight variation of a calcification from previous mammograms. The first thing that I thought was, "Thank God my children are adults (26 and 23 years old) who can take care of themselves and will be able to cope intellectually, if not emotionally." Having worked in the hectic world of television and being

president and/or board member of several community and national volunteer organizations, I felt confident that I would have the emotional strength and brains to deal with this bump in the road of my life.
(Helen B. Greenleaf)

My tumor was found by my primary care physician's nurse practitioner, herself a breast cancer survivor. I knew as soon as she found it that it was cancer. I had no idea it was there. I am a Registered Nurse, working as a case manager. Worked out at the local gym three days per week and walked an average of two miles daily. Low fat diet. First reaction? I was scared to death. My mother and sister had died of colon cancer and I figured that would be my fate, not breast cancer.
(Peggy Scott, Waldorf, MD, diagnosed in 2002 at age 46)

A health care manager with low-fat, no-red-meat diet for 15+ years. Nonsmoker and exercised 3-4 times a week for 15 years. No family history of breast cancer. I found the lump on breast self-exam after some slight discomfort and dimpling. My mammogram was negative, but an ultrasound detected the mass and the core biopsy showed malignancy. My initial reaction was fear, and I just wanted it out of my body.
(Alicia, diagnosed in 2001 at age 41)

A routine mammogram at age 56 found suspicious cells requiring a biopsy. I accepted the news with surprising calmness, partly because I had been reading about breast cancer for years and figured my luck could run out any day. I was so wrapped up in my home-based business at the time that I didn't have time to get emotional. My immediate concern was not the salvation of my breast, but of my business schedule and whether I'd lose my hair.
(Barbara Brabec)

The lump was not cancerous but it drove me to have the mammograms. I had calcifications, which can not be felt but were detected by the mammograms. The calcifications were cancerous.
(Donna Tremblay, diagnosed in 1992 at age 33, recurrence in 1996)

A research microbiologist, married with two daughters ages 3 and 6, diagnosed at age 37. My left breast was painful at times. A mammogram revealed calcifications. The doctor said to come back in one year. About 6 months later I discovered a pea-size lump, like a pebble, very hard, in my left breast while performing BSE in the shower—which by the way seems to be the best place to perform them. A fine needle biopsy confirmed the cancer. I was practically hysterical, and I couldn't even listen to details about surgery and drainage tubes. I was so glad that my husband was with me to comfort me as well as get all the information. I felt like I was walking around in such a fog for a very long time.

(Carolyn S. Olson, diagnosed at age 37)

I was diagnosed in 2001 at age 57. I don't believe my work stress caused my cancer, but it most certainly contributed. Sometimes I feel like a rubber band, stretched to the limit. I deprived myself of sleep, ate badly, didn't exercise, and I smoked, drank too much coffee and generally put everyone else before myself. I have paid a very high price for my follies. I let life get in the way of caring for the person who is the most important to me—myself. A mammogram fourteen months earlier showed no signs, and I was told I don't need another one for at least two years. These tests are vital to saving lives. It's always about money and cutting costs. A biopsy came back negative but the lump, removed by a lumpectomy, showed a malignant tumor. Being up to my rear in alligators on occasion certainly has its own stressors, and it took me a long time to learn to say the magic word "no." It was an eternity before my husband came home. Even though the words were unspoken I know we were both thinking I would die. The children, too, thought I was going to die. A pathology report then showed that the margins were not clean, and I needed a radical mastectomy.

(Virginia, diagnosed in 2001 at age 57)

At age 37, I felt my right breast was somehow changing, and it felt like a "muscle" in the front part of the breast. Because I was young, had never smoked and did not seem in general to be at risk with no breast cancer in the family, my gynecologist said my breast was made like that. For a year and a half I kept touching my "muscle" and if I had second thoughts I always remembered my gyno words that it was "my breast was made like that." So I felt stupidly reassured. The funny thing is that I had always claimed that I was a very well informed person that cannot be fooled easily and yet... I went again to see my gynecologist when I was 39. The reason of my visit was not the breast, but I asked the doctor to check it "even though I knew that my breast was made like that." This time, he sent me for a mammogram. The tumor was more than 5 cm and cancerous. The surgeon asked me how on earth I had such a huge cancer and he hoped it had not spread. My world ended that day. I have no words to express the despair and the horrendous sinking feeling that I experienced. Something strange happened; I felt reborn and ready to fight. I am not a very positive person, quite the opposite. Nevertheless, that instant of change in my perception of the situation was quite remarkable. I had never experienced anything like that before.

(Elisa)

High stress job with the Federal Government, involving a lot of traveling. Active lifestyle, walked a lot, usually ate well. Felt a lump at age 62. I went to see a doctor and was told that it was nothing and to go home and not to worry. When I got home, I did worry and the next morning phoned the office to request a mammogram. I was met with a hostile response. I would stress that anyone with a lump should insist on a mammogram and not be intimidated by either the staff or the medical professionals, no matter how rude they may be. I had a partial mastectomy with axillary node dissection and sentinel lymph node biopsy. First reaction was disbelief and denial. I phoned my friend, sobbing, saying I was going to die and made her promise to take my cats for me.

(Sharron, diagnosed in 2002 at age 62)

Registered nurse, diagnosed in 2002 at age 47. It started as a thickening, but mammograms were negative for 8-10 years. Ultrasound signaled "fibrous" and I finally persuaded a surgeon to biopsy the lump. It felt like a long thin pencil with a tiny bead on the end, and I had "peau d'orange" skin markings (dimpling).

(Yvette, Victoria, BC, diagnosed in 2002 at age 47)

Married with two sons, a teacher of languages, diagnosed in 1999 at age 45. I was papering a room in my house and ran into the ladder with my right breast. It hurt so much, but I forgot about it. A month later, I felt my breast was as hard as a stone and I panicked. I have a lump of 5-7 cm.

When an oncologist does a biopsy, she starts telling me about cancer, chemotherapy, radiation… Lying there, I feel that the tears fall from my eyes right on the table. Biopsy results bring bad news. I have no feelings, I have no thoughts. I just sit there in a kind of empty hole. And I think, "If I do not move, if I sit still, time will stop and things won't get worse." When I went to see a gynecologist just two months earlier, everything had been all right and then I have such a huge lump!

(Annemie D'haveloose, Belgium, diagnosed in 1999 at age 45)

Married with three children and a Labrador, diagnosed at age 44. A nurse in anesthesiology, worked with cancer patients and in cancer research. I had just lost five kg (11 lbs.) to feel good about myself when I discovered a small lump in my right breast. There was breast cancer in my family, but they were all old ladies so I had no worries. But the tests revealed cancer. We gathered our three children and told them. Our son, age 12, spoke for all three. He wanted to know if I would die, and we had to promise that whatever news we would receive, good or bad, they had to be first to know. They all wanted a cell phone so they could call me at any time, and my little daughter jumped up and wanted her ear pierced. She got her ears pierced and five cell phones were bought.

(Karen Lisa Hilsted, Denmark)

A registered dental hygienist for 18 years, lead a clean life, low-fat diet. I was 39 years old in 1995. Our new puppy woke me up. I had an area in between my breasts that needed to be scratched. I felt a lump, like I was palpating a tangerine wedge.

(Kristina, diagnosed in 1995 at age 39)

I was 26 and 3 months away from my Cinderella wedding when I found a lump in my left breast. I found the lump myself because it was painful. At first I thought it was a pulled muscle from lifting weights. I went to the National Race for the Cure in DC (before diagnosis); they had the display of a breast with "lumps" in it so you could feel what you should look for in a breast self exam. Until you feel something, you really don't know what you are looking for. What I felt in that fake breast that day felt a lot like what I was feeling in my own breast.

(Julie)

Dealing With the Medical System

Doctors, appointments, hospitals, what makes a good patient

It is a sheer waste of time and soul-power to imagine what I would do if things were different. They are not different. (Frank Crane)

It was vital for me to find doctors I liked and trusted to aid in my recovery. I felt my surgeon wanted me to survive, and that gave me strength. Without being pushy, she guided me through my options with honesty and kindness. She saw the rapport I had with my children, and she treated me as a person and not just a patient. When I had a core biopsy, my daughter was holding my hand and my surgeon showed us both how to examine woman's breasts and what a cancerous tumor feels like compared to a fatty deposit, since I had both.

Clinical trials: Studies of new treatments are known as clinical trials. Instead of a standard treatment, you might be offered an option of participating in such a study. Get fully informed about potential benefits and drawbacks. Take your time before deciding, so you are comfortable with your decision. Find a doctor you trust and get a second opinion if you are unsure.

What makes a good doctor is one who cares, who tells the truth in a compassionate way and does not make the patient feel that she is only one of many.

(Dr. Barry J. Barclay, St. Albert, AB, lost his wife to breast cancer)

WHAT MAKES A GOOD PATIENT

Be on time for appointments but be prepared to wait. (Donate your old magazines to the hospital waiting rooms.)

Prepare relevant, straightforward questions before appointments. Take a tape recorder to the appointments or a friend for moral support and to make sure you won't misunderstand or forget anything.

Write down the answers to your questions.

Try booking the first appointment of the morning or after lunch in case more tests are needed. The doctor will be less rushed and might take more time with you.

Learn the language of your type of breast cancer to better understand the terminology used.

The time between my surgery and seeing an oncologist was very stressful and took over four weeks. I spent that time sitting by the phone waiting for a call. Finally I cracked and sent my husband to the hospital to plead my case. It seems the hospital had lost my file and was overworked. Thanks to a kind secretary, a compassionate oncologist squeezed me into his busy schedule.

(Lorraine Zakaib, Kirkland, QC, diagnosed in 2002 at age 49)

My doctors are great. They listen to all my questions, give me resources and their support office people made my care as smooth as possible. I decided to participate in a clinical trial by asking my doctor lots of questions. I spoke to others who had gone through cancer. Research is important and necessary, and I decided that the big picture would be that my participation might help in future treatment.

(Deborah, diagnosed in 2002 at age 46)

I decided that I wanted a mastectomy, because I could live without a breast but I could not live with cancer. My oncologist was so thorough and answered all my questions. He arranged for me to see a surgeon, who was my angel of mercy and incredible in the way she explained everything to me, before, during, and after. And then along came a plastic surgeon that was the icing on the cake. I opted for immediate reconstruction and so he did a TRAM flap at the same time. I was so very pleased to be able to wake from surgery feeling whole. Upon returning home, I hooked up with our local physiotherapist. She opened her studio to me and took a great interest in helping me regain my arm movement. She was instrumental in my recovery and we remain very close friends.

(Marylynn)

I chose standard treatment, because I didn't want to do clinical trials. My doctor wasn't happy with my choice.

(psh)

Because I work in a hospital and know oncologists and others working with cancer patients, I was able to quickly move through the medical system. What slowed me down the most was getting approvals from my insurance company, and this can be very frustrating!

(Joni)

I started a journal right at the beginning of it all, and this was invaluable. It filled up very quickly with appointment details, addresses, phone numbers, questions for me to ask the doctors, answers they gave me, as well as being a place for me to write down my feelings during the interminable waits for appointments and treatments.

(Judith Quinlan, diagnosed in 2001 at age 52)

My oncologist was excellent and encouraged me to learn as much as possible. This helped me and my family get a handle on things and become more rational. It also made me an educated consumer when I went for a second opinion. My biggest problem was my husband's fear that I was dying. It took him months to deal with this, and it seriously affected his mental and physical health. Knowledge made me a

Ideally, to make it easier for everyone, you'll find the medical team you like and trust.

***

Seek support from family and friends, but also from other women that have had the experience.

***

Be honest and proactive, in touch with your emotions and needs, and participate fully in the decisions about surgery and treatments.

***

Listen attentively to what the doctor is saying about the options and possible side effects, how the surgery and treatments will be performed, and what you should expect.

***

Take personal responsibility for your own health and cooperate with the doctor.

***

Do not self-diagnose or get scared after surfing the Internet, but gather relevant questions. Every case is different. Only your own doctor can tell you about your cancer.

***

better patient, and I knew the relevant questions to ask to take an active role in my treatment.

(Anonymous)

I chose the doctor I did because, after looking at their experience and skills, she treated me like a person, not a disease. I think a good patient is someone who is respectful but advocates for what she needs. I asked many questions but I always wrote them down and tried to be aware of the doctor's time.

(Lorraine Langdon-Hull)

My oncologist was amazing. He took the time needed to answer all my questions and never made me feel rushed. I prepared my questions and wrote them in a book, which I took with me to all the appointments. I also read about the various treatments and educated myself on breast cancer.

(Debbie Giroux, Langley, BC)

A good patient is someone who asks a lot of questions and is a pain in the butt. I wanted to make sure that the doctors knew me as Jacqui and not just a number.

(Jacqui, Courtenay, BC, diagnosed in 2002 at age 38)

I liked my doctor. He made me feel like we could beat this, and he kept telling me I was a real trooper.

(Linda Bryngelson, New Brighton, MN)

My cancer had spread so it was no longer curable, but it was treatable. One of the things I found useful after diagnosis was a book my surgeon gave me. It explained about the various types of breast cancer and how the disease develops and proceeds. It also talked about treatment options and communicating with your doctors. I found after reading the book that I had many questions.

(Kathy Reeve, North Vancouver, BC, diagnosed in 2000 at age 32)

I chose to go on a clinical trial. I decided quickly because I was scared. By reading Dr. Susan Love's Breast Book I knew that only 1-4% of all breasts cancers were this type (inflammatory) and that I wanted to take every chance I was given to survive. What makes a good doctor? I had more than 26! There are so many aspects. My oncologist has fingers I trust and is as bright as can be. My surgeon did an excellent job slicing off my breast and half of my underarm leaving me a thin scar and a total range of motion. Good doctors have bounce. They listen. They speak directly. They keep doing their job. They might not always be polite or on time, but they do know what they are doing and communicate when necessary in an immediate fashion.

(Maria Hindmarch)

I went alone to all my treatments. It was my choice. I wanted to make myself strong and not feel dependent on anyone. I think my treatment would have been much smoother had I gone to a comprehensive cancer center. As it was, the radiology department was associated with one hospital, my surgeon with another, and my oncologist with a third. The surgeon referred me to one oncologist but a book I read strongly recommends getting a second opinion. I did get that second opinion and it changed my whole approach to treatment (no chemo). However,

Be your own assertive advocate, yet patient and understanding with your doctors and the staff. They are often overworked and stressed. You can help them do their best and more, sometimes in very difficult circumstances. You can help them help you.

Research the doctors and find the right medical team. Check references and get referrals to feel empowered about your choices, or get someone else do this for you.

Get a second or third opinion if needed.

Your pharmacist will provide accurate and useful information about medications and side effects. They are highly educated, helpful, and unbiased.

Tell your doctors everything out of the ordinary during treatments. Keep notes so you won't forget. They will recognize the red flags that might signal possible complications.

For scheduled tests, ask in advance if you are allowed to eat or, if fasting, drink water in case they forget to tell you.

Involve your doctor to get the appointments sooner and to get test results. Ideally you will have the same doctor all the time who is familiar with the whole situation. If you must change doctors, provide copies of your tests and treatments to the new team.

Help your doctors and nurses to get to know you on a personal level. This makes the treatments more pleasant for both parties.

"Too young" is not a diagnosis.

Research factual, up-to-date information and options on your type of cancer at the hospital library, breast health centers, the Internet, support groups, and from hotlines. See web sites and books on pages 218-219.

choosing the second oncologist who wasn't part of the original team complicated things for me. My surgeon gave me a videotape of the sentinel node procedure. That helped calm the fear of the "unknown." I love my oncologist. I feel he treats each patient individually and cares about the psychological toll that a breast cancer diagnosis takes. He tape-records the initial consultation and gives his patients the tape. That way when one returns home and is totally confused, one can play the tape back as a reminder of what was said.

(Rita, Palos Verdes, CA)

It took great effort to proceed through the consults and further tests, to continue working throughout, and to do research to educate myself on my situation and the medical terminology and to examine each treatment option to decide what was best. I felt completely overwhelmed and scared of making the wrong decision because of the limited time I had to learn everything. The chaos only calmed down when I decided upon a treatment facility, oncologist, surgeon, and treatment options, and the dates were set to start.

(Dikla, North Hollywood, CA)

I want a doctor to tell me what I need to know and not throw numbers and percentages at me.

(Julie Austin, Little Rock, AR, diagnosed in 2000 at age 30)

The first surgeon misread the pathology report and wanted to perform a double mastectomy. An oncologist told me the test results were misread and I needed no further surgery other than a lymph node biopsy. Another surgeon also misread the report. I finally saw a renowned breast cancer surgeon for referral. My surgeon there was wonderful. He performed the sentinel node biopsy. The cancer had not spread to my lymph nodes. I cried tears of joy and was relieved.

(Stephanie)

I trusted initial providers and had excellent care. I also had good health coverage, quite a blessing. My chemo doctor was smart and up-to-date but barely human. I left his care as soon as chemo was over and switched to an herbalist/oncologist for all follow-up care. My vascular surgeon, a woman, was meticulously careful with the nerves so that they were spared. I had a plastic surgeon during mastectomy who put in an inflatable prosthesis in preparation for eventual reconstruction. The prosthesis was awful.

(Suzanna Stinnett)

After my biopsy, my surgeon came in to tell me the tumor was malignant. He said that he was sure I'd be fine and that I'd live to be 90, which cheered me up a little.

(Leslie, Springfield, VA)

"Too young" is not a diagnosis. Follow up with your doctor if you have a lump that grows.

(Johnna Fielder)

A good doctor has compassion. I don't think doctors should give a prognosis for survival time. It varies for every individual person. While I see reason for giving some idea of what to expect, being made to believe you only have a certain amount of time left to live is limiting.

(Marie, Co. Mayo, Ireland, diagnosed in 1987, recurrence 13 years later)

When I was diagnosed, I asked the surgeon if I could set up informational meetings with an oncologist, radiologist, and reconstruction surgeon, and that I wanted to see a chemo session. The surgeon was astonished and his exact words were, "Usually our patients don't want that much information and find it overwhelming." I answered him by saying that I've already been told I had cancer, and did he think I couldn't take it? I was trained as a reporter, so my natural instinct was to get all the facts on the story and then form my own conclusions. I was very, very lucky. My father is a departmental head for a major medical college and I had access to the best of the best in their fields for second opinions.

(Mary Schmidt)

There was no question in my mind that my surgeon was the top in his field and my trust in him was implicit. As far as the oncologists, let's just say that I'm on my 3rd oncologist. The first one told me that I asked too many questions (wouldn't you if you had been diagnosed with cancer?), and my second one spent under 90 seconds with me for each examination. The nurses were kind though, and they got me through the wretched chemotherapy. I am now with my 3rd oncologist (a woman) and I feel as though I've hit the jackpot. The best advice I can give anyone is to be positive. The way you go through the treatment will follow.

(Dawn, North Hollywood, CA, diagnosed in 2001 at age 47)

I told the doctor that I could not, and would not wait and that I needed the surgery done ASAP—not to mention the fact that I had a family vacation planned two days post-op and I was not going to miss it. I spend at least a week every summer with my brother, sister-in-law and three nephews in a cabin in northern Wisconsin, and I truly believed that the beginning of my road to recovery would be best started with them.

(Cindy, Cedarburg, WI, diagnosed at age 41)

My doctor was wonderful! Although the head of surgery at a large metropolitan hospital, he took the time to answer all my questions both before and after the surgery and during my follow-up appointments. I think a good patient must become her own advocate and do research and ask questions that will make the doctor think and respond. This sets up a rapport that makes you an individual in the doctor's eyes and not just another patient.

(Sherry Gaffney, diagnosed in 1989 at age 47)

A local oncologist was very presumptuous about the results and treatment based on my age. He said I wouldn't be able to do hormone therapy because my cancer wouldn't be estrogen receptor positive, but in fact I did end up being positive. The next clue that I needed a second opinion was when he told me to cancel my wedding. I did get a second opinion at a Cancer Center in the city, and they were wonderful. I felt very comfortable with them. They gave me a recommendation about my treatment based on facts and never assumed anything based on my age. I did fine throughout the process. I think in a lot of cases I didn't realize really how serious this all was, and I was in a lot of ways lucky that I had my wedding to look forward to. When you are in a whirlwind of doctors and treatments and just trying to save up some energy to spend with a new spouse, there's no time to stop and think beyond what is happening at the moment. When you stop the chemo and radiation and only see doctors every three months, you start dealing with the reality of it all and what happens next. The worst part about dealing with the medical system is the insurance company and following exactly the right rules to get the coverage you deserve. Keep all the documentation of bills, insurance papers, copies of referrals, and notes of when you called and who you talked to. If you don't have the energy or organizational skills to do this, find someone who can help you. It will make things easier. The last thing you need to worry about is insurance and paying the bills.

(Julie, diagnosed at age 26)

My husband, who is a doctor, usually does not give up but this time he did. His colleague who was a breast surgeon couldn't/wouldn't help. So I sent my husband over to some of our very good friends, and I went to an old friend who is also a doctor. I made a few phone calls and everything was planned before I went to bed that night. I was operated seven days later. I had chemo and radiation at the same ward I had worked for several years. I felt that they looked at me more like a colleague and a friend, and this made me feel very safe.

(Karen Lisa Hilsted, Denmark)

If you feel a lump or see any change in your breast, insist on a biopsy. Some doctors will say, "Let's wait awhile and keep an eye on it," but don't settle for that, get it attended to now.

(Chris Lengert, Campbell River, BC, diagnosed in 1996 at age 52)

A good patient pushes past the fear and finds out everything she can about the disease and treatment options. She isn't afraid to ask questions. I kept a notebook for questions and answers, and a multi-pocket portfolio with sections for appointments, chemo and radiation information, insurance info, perks from friends, receipts, etc.

(Alicia)

I basically had two days to decide what to do. The first day I spent washing windows and ignoring the situation. The second day I contacted the Cancer Society breast cancer volunteer (who's a friend) and we met for lunch and talked about it. My doctor is compassionate, caring and I felt I had known him forever.

(Cheryl Otting, Elkford, BC, diagnosed in 2002 at age 53)

I had a lumpectomy. Two years later I had a rash and a new lump soon after. I fear that cancer was already in my lymph nodes two years before, but because they didn't check, it spread. I was very, very angry and disillusioned with the medical community.

(Heather Resnick, Thornhill, ON, diagnosed in 1997 at age 43, recurrence in 1999)

I had access to a leading breast cancer oncologist, a fabulous oncology breast surgeon, and an incredible plastic surgeon. I think everyone should get the best possible medical care that is available and accessible and not make any assumptions. One of the best places to get this information is from a support group.

(Debbie Peake)

Take someone you trust to all appointments with you. Take notes and ask questions. If your doctor doesn't want to answer them or you don't feel that he/she is being honest with you, find someone else. You cannot bury your head under a rock, as this is something you have to face head on. Learn the terminology and facts about what you are facing right now, but don't get too far ahead of yourself. I chose a clinical trial because I want my cancer to mean something to those that will come behind me. I am scared to death that my daughters might have to fight this themselves one day.

(Peggy Scott, Waldorf, MD, diagnosed in 2002 at age 46)

The medical system was excellent. Small hospitals can be wonderful! My surgeon said to be safe there really was no choice but a modified radical mastectomy. I was happy to agree.

(Joan Fox, Victoria, BC)

My medical center has a wonderful program for breast cancer. It is a group diagnosis, and you meet with all your "new friends" individually on one day. They meet and discuss options and come to a group conclusion. I have been phoned by my surgeon three times to tell me the diagnosis of the biopsy and the surgery, by the radiation oncologist, and by psychologist. I call the radiation department my tanning salon.

(Toni)

I was treated in a small hospital (with the quality of a university hospital), in the "one day" department for oncology. I have been very lucky because I was treated as a person, not as a number. A good doctor to me is one who tells you the truth immediately and one who explains to you what's going to happen next. "You have cancer," is very hard to hear, but at least it is clear. You have to trust the doctors and do what they tell you. Ask all the possible questions so that there are no doubts left in your head. That's what a good patient is, in my opinion—no dealing with doubts and half-truths. Stick to the truth, and use all the energy for positive fight.

(Annemie D'haveloose, Belgium , diagnosed in 1999 at age 45)

My oncologist was very intelligent and good at spewing stats and numbers but lacked a humanitarian touch. She was dogmatic whereas the patient needs to feel she has some control or choices. It was a "do this or else" attitude and that was very disempowering.

(Yvette, Victoria, BC, diagnosed in 2002 at age 47)

You have to look at each situation individually and let the doctors help you with the decision, but basically you must choose what will be done to your body. Some people can discuss things better than others, so take someone with you who is strong and supportive so as not to zap your energies. It's good to talk to someone going through this even as early as just being diagnosed. Ask for copies of all tests. I wish I had known that after age 50 you can have a mammogram annually. Get a second opinion if you want it even if it delays the treatment; you will feel better mentally. It is your body.

(Penny)

If I learned one thing about breast cancer from all of this, I learned how important it is to do your monthly breast exams. That is how I found my lump, and there was no doubt in my mind that the "golf ball" that I was feeling did not belong there. The annual mammogram is important too, but in my case, the mammogram that I had following the discovery of the lump showed nothing. Nothing! And my tumor was rather large. I am thankful that, despite the results of the mammogram, the medical personnel were proactive and immediately recommended seeing a surgeon. The rest is history.

(Debbie Garrett)

Friends brought me books on cancer, the hospital gave me information, and I researched breast cancer on the Internet. I was consumed with this wealth of information.

(Sheryl)

A biopsy came back negative, but the lump, removed by a lumpectomy, showed a malignant tumor. How could a negative diagnosis have turned into this nightmare? It was eerie, surreal. Margins were not clean so I had a radical mastectomy. Facing reality is a very difficult thing. Hugs from the nursing staff worked magic. The oncologist was brusque but thorough. I'm glad he wasn't a wishy-washy kind of person. He was straight to the point and had a "get on with it" attitude. That helped me stay strong. Warm and fuzzy, I didn't need.

(Virginia, diagnosed in 2001 at age 57)

I felt sorry for myself, living away from any family member and being by myself in rural southwestern Indiana. My arm swelled a lot and it was quite uncomfortable so I had to have the fluid aspirated. The doctor's assistant was born to be a nurse. My surgeon was a younger man but very personable. He did not mind sharing information about his family so I got to know him somewhat on a personal level, which was important to me. I even got to know about his assistant's dogs and other things, and that made them both seem more like regular people, a trait that I particularly appreciated. Within three weeks I was back to work because that made me feel like I was getting better and not letting this disease get me down.

(Joy McCarthy-Sessing)

That was an excruciating decision: Should I go for the standard treatment or the clinical trial? After researching on the Internet, and even consulting with statisticians about the significance of some early results, I took the decision of taking the standard treatment.

(Elisa)

My first oncologist was very research- and not people-oriented. He strongly recommended that I sign on to a clinical trial and implied that I would get better follow-up if I were on the study. I wanted to make an informed decision but did not know where to turn. I called the oncology nurse and asked her where I could get more information and she said, "You don't need any more information than what the doctor has already given you." I found out months later (after the decision had been painstakingly made) that there was a library right in the oncology department, with tons of books and literature on breast cancer. The Quebec Cancer Foundation sent a stack of information. I had second and third opinions and chose not to participate in the study.

(Donna Tremblay, diagnosed in 1992 at age 33, recurrence in 1996)

Surgeries

Lumpectomy, mastectomy, reconstruction, regaining arm movement

There is no good arguing with the inevitable. The only argument available with the east wind is to put on your overcoat. (James Russell Lowell)

I had never paid much attention to my breasts. With envy, I now noticed breasts everywhere, young and old in all sizes, beautiful, soft, symmetric, and feminine. But the cancer was growing inside me, and a mastectomy was inevitable and urgent. My daughter put it in a comforting perspective by saying, "Luckily you can still see and walk and read and write your books without a breast." I had felt exhausted both mentally and physically for a while so when I was diagnosed, the treatments gave me a good excuse to rest for a few months.

The possibility of a reconstruction, a serious elective surgery, comforted me initially, and I met women with good results. But now, five years later, I still have not done it, and with each passing year it seems less important. I keep postponing it and might never find time, need, or courage to do it. Well, I might reconsider it if they can plant a cell in me that will grow a new breast without pain or complications and with guaranteed results.

In the hospital one day, while waiting for my pre-op tests, another patient who had never regained her full arm movement repeatedly urged me to do the exercises consistently and immediately after surgery. I wish I could thank her now.

To make things easier for chemo injections and for drawing blood, they installed a port-a-cath near my collarbone due to my weak veins. It was removed a few months after chemo ended.

Lumpectomy

After lumpectomy, my breast was heavy and swollen and I couldn't wear a bra so I tied a long strip of gauze into a handy breast-sling. I did not have drains but a painless procedure of aspirating the accumulated liquid three times at the hospital. Later, only a seamless bra without underwire was comfortable enough. Even now, two years later, underwire bras press on my scar tissue and hurt.

(Maarit)

I have small breasts so even the lumpectomy was disfiguring. I have a hard time finding bras that fit correctly.

(Alicia)

The worst news, a week after lumpectomy, was that they didn't get clean margins around the tumor. I was devastated. I thought, "You didn't kill me the first time so you're going to give it another shot." My incision was healing beautifully and I wanted to get on with the rest of it. But I bit the bullet and went back. For the first time since the kids were born my husband and I went to the zoo and county fair like we were dating again. Surgery loomed like an island and I was stranded at sea. I both welcomed and feared it. The worst part was the pre-op insertion of two wires (tumor markers). This was done on the ultrasound table under local anesthesia. Then I walked down the hall with the two wires sticking out of my breast about six inches feeling like I was receiving AM and FM

CLOTHING

Baggy comfort clothing for several weeks. Soft, loose, comfortable, 100% cotton, button-down clothing. Big shirts, sweats or loose-fitting pants with elastic waist, housecoat, wraparound robe or top. A soft, comfortable pair of pajamas (without scratchy lace). Jogging pants and a button-down or zippered shirt and sweaters larger than usual. A Hawaiian muumuu.

DRAINS

If you have drain tubes, pin them to your clothes to keep pulling on your skin, or slip them into your pockets/fanny pack.

BRA TIPS

A sports bra with front hooks, or a seamless bra (no underwires). After lumpectomy, your breast might be swollen and heavy and you might need a bigger bra for a while. If necessary, make a sling to support your breast while recovering.

BREAST ENHANCERS

If needed after a lumpectomy, breast enhancers are available in several shapes, at the mastectomy boutique, to fill out your bra.

PROSTHESES

Some women find a prosthesis heavy, hot, and uncomfortable, but it works for balance. A breast can weigh a lot. Mastectomy boutiques have lightweight prostheses, stick-ons, prosthesis bras, swimsuit prostheses, camisoles with hidden pockets, and bras with extended lower section for comfort.

OTHER OPTIONS

Go braless, layer clothing, wear big shirt or scarf for camouflage. Fill your bra with shoulder pads. Make a lightweight pouch filled with fluffy stuffing, pin to bra or camisole under another shirt for a soft mound. Try a loose cardigan, jacket or vest with a hidden inside pocket to pad if needed.

radio. Then ouch they did a mammogram with the wires in—fun, fun, fun. The site healed quickly. The underarm area was another story. Besides numbness, one night I was awakened by shooting pains and needed pain medication to get through it. This is from someone who rarely takes an aspirin.

(Diane Dorman)

After a lumpectomy, I had to have a second surgery as they did not have clean margins. It was very easy to recover from. I did not require a prosthesis; it is amazing how the breast fills in naturally. Sometimes while doing the exercises I could hear water sloshing and it was the fluid in my breast. It does eventually get absorbed. I used only extra-strength acetaminophen and sometimes after exercise would take one. Mostly I drank herbal tea, and I listened to relaxing music while taking deep breaths. Even a lumpectomy can leave you feeling apprehensive. Daily positive thinking can help.

(Penny)

Being as young as I am, I was concerned how my breast would look afterwards. I was happy to find that my breast was still quite "whole" once it healed. The pain was really not too bad after the first couple of days. A soft comfy bra is a very good thing.

(Jennifer, diagnosed in 2001 at age 27)

The stereoscopic biopsy was very nice. The nurse even massaged me with scents and there was pleasant music! Calcifications are very small and impossible to see except with biopsy after the surgery. I had two lumpectomies and then had to do a third surgery, this time a mastectomy. I read Dr. Susan Love's Breast Book a lot, always needing to read new chapters after each call from the doctor.

(S.R., Columbus, OH)

I had the standard treatments with chemo, radiation and a lumpectomy in between. I was told that I might have some pain and to give it three years. Sure enough, in three years the pain was gone. I think it was a good thing to know.

(Esther Matsubuchi, North Vancouver, BC)

I was surprised at how little discomfort I had after the lumpectomy. I was back at work the following week but could have gone sooner. I found that it was important to massage the breast as it helped to keep adhesions from forming. I didn't do this soon enough on a later excisional biopsy in the same area, and now my depression is more noticeable because it is attached to the chest muscle.

(Rita, Palos Verdes, CA)

I have not used a prosthesis, and I can't tell the difference between my breasts unless I really look carefully. The worst part was the anticipation. The other difficult part for me was having to go with my son to the pre-surgical appointment so he could learn how to deal with the drain if I needed one, which I didn't. He's a good guy, and he made jokes throughout the appointment to keep it light. I wore a short-sleeved heavy-knit shirt that buttoned down the front when I came home from the hospital, which was the same afternoon that I had my lumpectomy. Selecting something roomy and

COLD BREAST

Drinking cold water can make your breast suddenly very cold. Swimming can give you cramps and pain. It is normal and a temporary discomfort after surgery and radiation.

RESTING AFTER

Lots of pillows at night are comfortable. For the first few nights, a recliner is a safe comfort zone for resting, sleeping, napping, reading, dreaming, contemplating your life. You'll feel more mobile and comfortable than in a bed, especially after a mastectomy. Electric recliner helps after reconstruction.

DON'T GO HOME ALONE

You might feel sad, lonely, and unprepared when you leave the hospital so arrange for someone to bring you home. If family or friends are not available, ask someone in the support group to accompany you and get you settled.

DRAINS

If you come home with drains (to suction and collect fluid from surgical area), have a nurse show and explain to you how to empty them and measure the amount of liquid in them. Get written instructions. When showering is allowed, pin the drains to something tied around your body or neck such as a scarf, pantyhose, dental floss, or elastic, so your arms are free and the drains won't pull your skin.

REGAINING FULL ARM MOVEMENT AND AVOIDING FROZEN SHOULDER

Start exercising your arm right away even though it will hurt. You are not harming your scar by exercising; you are harming yourself if you don't. Be vigilant and persistent. Ask for written instructions or a video of exercises to perform after surgery. In some hospitals, volunteers will demonstrate the exercises. Keep moving, do not baby your arm. A physiotherapist is able to help you if needed.

fairly dark that I could button myself was a real challenge. I live in Southern California and it was very hot. I just wanted to be comfortable.

(Rita, Santa Clarita, CA)

My breast deflated a bit and had a dent where the scar was, but a year later the breast has filled out almost entirely. I am very happy with the physical form results. The most uncomfortable part after the surgery was dealing with the drains.

(Dikla, North Hollywood, CA)

I had a lumpectomy with an axillary node dissection. My underarm was very sore and no one had prepared me for this. My arm was stuck to my side. I could barely drive my car and function properly. Since my margins were not clean, it was necessary to remove more tissue. This time I was awake. It was a frightening experience to hear and feel what was happening.

(Lorraine Zakaib, Kirkland, QC, diagnosed in 2002 at age 49)

The doctor who removed my tumor thought he was removing a cyst. He was a plastic surgeon and took very little tissue, yet he obtained clear margins around the tumor. There was no scarring and no pain, and only a local anesthetic was used.

(Stephanie)

I have no prosthesis. My arm that had the lymph nodes removed will never be the same. It will always be weaker than the other one, but I sure can live with that. That arm also gets tired faster than the other one.

(Joy McCarthy-Sessing)

After two cancers in the same place, I wear a small balance prosthesis in the bottom of my bra.

(Bev Parker, Naperville, IL, diagnosed in 1985 at age 40, recurrence in 2001)

The best advice I have is try not to baby the arm once the incision is healed. I got a massage about 3 weeks post-op, highly recommended. The incision is healed and the range should start to come back in the arm. A massage can take care of many of life's problems.

(Cindy, Cedarburg, WI, diagnosed at age 41)

No pain or discomfort! I would have liked surgery to leave both breasts looking the same but truthfully, in time, it stopped bothering me.

(Laura)

Not that much tissue, it just looks like a small bite was taken out! No prosthesis needed, but I do feel more comfortable in padded bras and swimsuits with a soft cup bra in them, especially because my nipple doesn't face forward anymore. Pain is almost daily, but you just learn what feels good and what doesn't.

(Peggy Scott, Waldorf, MD, diagnosed in 2002 at age 46)

I wear a bathing suit prosthesis, just need a little something to give my breast some shape. I had no discomfort or pain.

(Chris Lengert, Campbell River, BC, diagnosed in 1996 at age 52)

I never thought of a mastectomy because my cancer had already metastasized. All through life I felt my breasts were too small. However I remember looking at my breasts in the mirror

---

EXERCISES TO REGAIN ARM MOVEMENT

Put on some nice music, keep moving, and massage your arm. Here are some good exercises to regain your arm movement.

---

1) Walk your fingers up the wall as high as you can, over and over, every day, repeatedly.

---

2) Lie on your back, raise your arms and bring them back over your head.

---

3) As soon as you are allowed, stretch in a warm shower so your muscles are relaxed and your scar won't hurt so much.

---

4) Standing, lift your arms to your sides as high as you can, hold until you no longer feel the pain, about 20 seconds, and lift the arms an inch higher, hold again, and so on. Repeat several times each day.

PAIN

You might feel pain with every little thing you do (burning sensation, brief acute stabbing pains, tingling, itchiness, numbness). Soften your breast and scar tissue gently with a warm shower, and massage it with cream to keep adhesions from forming. Months and even years after surgery you might feel tightness, stabbing pain, brief but severe and scary, with nerve endings coming back to life. Ask your doctor about every pain you feel. For backaches and muscle pain, wrap a heatbag around your waist (see page 91). Blast warm water on your scar with shower head set on massage for instant relief. Stretch. Massage. Try tiger balm, warm compresses, aspirin, hot showers, warm baths, and sauna.

NUMBNESS

Partial underarm numbness caused by lymph node dissection may last for years or forever.

after my ultrasound and thinking how perfect they were and that I should be happy with them. They served their purpose, as they allowed me to breast-feed my daughter. They didn't define me as a person, and they were exactly the size they were suppose to be. After surgery I wasn't too upset over the loss. After all I only lost a small part of my left breast, and it could have been worse. Now as I go on with my life I have some anxiety around my loss of part of my breast. I am single and it is something I would have to discuss if I were to pursue an intimate relationship with a man. This hasn't happened yet, but I think this is something I would struggle with. I do not need a prosthesis, and a padded bra can usually camouflage the missing area. I would like to get a prosthesis to wear with my bathing suit, as I am self-conscious. I found the pain after surgery bearable but became very nauseated from the medication, and that was hard to control. The drain I was sent home with caused me problems. I also found that my incision would leak at night, and I would wake up with a big wet spot and have to go to the hospital to have the dressing changed. *(Kathy Reeve, North Vancouver, BC, diagnosed in 2000 at age 32)*

I did not need reconstruction, but I do recommend a prosthesis to all women. For years I used several shoulder pads in my bras. It wasn't until last year that I requested a prosthesis from the Cancer Society. How dumb on my part! I believe every woman should feel good about herself and should definitely look into getting a prosthesis. What makes us look good, makes us feel good. I live a healthy good life, life that is full of exercise from swimming to walking. I am not ashamed about losing a portion of my breast and speak freely about it to those who ask. Life goes on and I want to partake of everything that is out there.

(Gwyn Ramsey)

My second surgeon, a woman, really respected my femininity by leaving only a tiny scar on my breast and virtually none under my arm. I thank her to this day for that beautiful job. Things healed up nicely, aided by my husband's rubbing Vitamin E oil into the scar every night for several months. This not only helped the skin, but also gave him something constructive to do to aid in my healing (instead of worrying), which was very important.

(Anonymous)

I had three lumpectomies total, all in the same breast. Now my breast is about half the size of the other one. I am not that big-breasted so I did not need a prosthesis. I thought the lumpectomies were very easy to recover from and really no big deal at all. I did have an axillary node dissection, and that was much tougher. I had a tube under my arm for ten days, and my underarm has just never been the same.

(Lorraine Langdon-Hull)

Mastectomy and reconstruction

Margins were not clear in the partial mastectomy so I had to go back for a total mastectomy. I had a saline implant as I was not a good candidate for the TRAM flap and did not want

TINGLY, ITCHY, NUMB UNDERARM AND SCAR

For a maddening itching in your scar area and under your numb arm, try blasting it with fairly hot water (shower head set on massage mode). Hot water relieves the tightness and pain in the scar and gives instant relief. Try rubbing it gently with a rough towel in shower. Cream or lotion, body powder, or cornstarch might help.

SCAR CARE

When the scar has healed, gently massage it with olive oil, Shea butter, sweet almond oil, Aloe Vera cream or gel, or Bag Balm. The redness and thickness of the scar will lessen over time.

PATIENCE

Take it one step at a time. Treatments are temporary. Things will get better.

Sidebar

HELP AFTER MAJOR SURGERY

Let others help, and tell them what you need. Have meals prepared ahead. You might not be able to drive for a while, so have someone take you around and run errands. Don't rush, give yourself time to heal. Do light chores to keep moving when you are up to it. Get someone to do the housework, or just let it wait.

BATHING AND BANDAGES AFTER MAJOR SURGERY

Consider having a bath chair and a lift bar for the bath. Use a no-slip tub mat. Have enough bandage supplies on hand, if needed.

TAKE PICTURES

Take pictures of yourself being bald and with your wig. Think of this as a different experience in your life.

PAMPER YOURSELF

Think of your own needs first. Allow yourself to become healthily egoistic.

---

the Dorsi flap. I did not have any regrets and really did not feel any remorse about losing part of my body, probably because there was so much cancer in it that I was glad to do whatever was necessary to rid my body of this hideous growth. To this date, I do not feel any remorse or regret over the loss of the breast. This could be in part due to my age (almost 64). I am content to live alone. If I do find a special person and they can not accept me as I am, they are not good enough for me.

(Sharron, diagnosed in 2002 at age 62)

Avoid listening to bad stories. The experience can be devastating if you let it. Have your pity party and move on.

(Johnna Fielder)

Be kind to yourself. If you feel like spending the day on the bed, do so. I asked about reconstruction and was told to deal with that later. My age, as well as some of the reconstruction problems my friends have had, helped make my decision to do nothing. I am still happy with my decision. I was 58 years old and my husband was very understanding. To this day I still wear a prosthesis and it hasn't fallen out yet, and the dog hasn't tried to eat it! Emotionally and physically I am completely content without my breast.

(Joan Fox, Victoria, BC)

I opted for a bilateral mastectomy with immediate reconstruction, which I did one month after this whole nightmare began. I was happy and it was helpful to wake up from surgery with "mounds" in the place of my breasts (at least I still had a cleavage). My oncologist suggested that I have my ovaries removed because of the strong family history of cancer. I was both sad and devastated, because I had seen what my sister had gone through and looked into the faces of my young sons and husband, who were all terrified. I had a combination saline and silicone implant. I did have to have my implants later removed and replaced (due to problems with the radiation) and I'm happy to say that I now have breasts complete with areolas and nipples. I don't mourn my breasts. They had fed my children, entertained my husband and rounded out (no pun intended) my sex life.

(Dawn, North Hollywood, CA, diagnosed in 2001 at age 47)

After two lumpectomies, the margins were still not clear so a mastectomy and simultaneous reconstruction followed. I did not experience a great amount of pain or discomfort. I practiced scar tissue massage regularly. I had my reconstruction at the same time as the mastectomy, and I have been very happy with the work of my surgeons. Right after I was told I need a mastectomy, I cried for about an hour, then dried my tears and tried to see the best way to get through that. I spent a lot of time in my garden, which I found very therapeutic.

(Dawn, Victoria, BC)

Regular mammograms did not show the cancer. The surgeon did MRI of both breasts, which found an additional tumor. Chemo was used before surgery to shrink the tumor and the lumpectomy was performed successfully with good cosmetic results. My surgeon just happened to take an extra piece of tissue at the end

MASSAGE

A massage or a visit to an osteopath can do wonders after all the invasive and painful treatments.

USE WHATEVER HELPS

Use humor, positive or even negative thinking, meditation, support, spirituality, journaling, chocolate, ice cream... to help you feel better.

MOVING ON

Avoid listening to bad stories. Have your pity party and move on.

NUTRITION

Fresh, nutritious food will restore your cells and your health, and will give you energy to cope and heal.

RECONSTRUCTION

Take your time to weigh all your options before you decide. Talk to others. Consult a reputable plastic surgeon. Get a second opinion. Consider the pros and cons. Be prepared for a lengthy recovery time.

---

of the guide wire. This biopsy determined more cancer. I opted for a bilateral mastectomy with implant reconstruction and did the full drill of nipples and tattoos, too. I then completed six more rounds of chemo. Nobody can tell you what it is like to remove your breast(s). There is a lot of input from your friends and family with, "Well, if I had breast cancer, I would…" Bottom line is they don't and can't relate to making your decision so unless their input is solicited, ignore it. If you have reconstruction at the same time as surgery, rent an electric lounge chair from a hospital supply company, since it will be difficult to lay down on your bed without assistance.

(Debbie Peake)

I opted for bilateral mastectomies with TRAM flap reconstruction after my second breast cancer. Because I had already had radiation on the left side, this was a good option for me. I also liked the idea of using my own tissue for the reconstruction. Although the recovery was difficult, I'm glad I made the decision I did and am happy with the results. I was glad my plastic surgeon was able to do the reconstruction at the same time as the mastectomies so I didn't have two major surgeries. I just had to go back later after chemo was finished to have nipple reconstruction, which was a simple surgery.

(Joni)

I had a fairly large lump removed. Three sides did not have clean borders so I had a full mastectomy and reconstruction surgery. I am starting to feel better although still get tired very easily.

(Debbie Giroux, Langley, B.C.)

The route to go into surgery is a very personal and of course emotional decision. My decision was fairly clear-cut from the start. I was determined to do as much as I could to eradicate the cancer. I chose a double mastectomy with reconstruction. My mother passed away at 43 years old from this disease. I was 13 years old. I hadn't even had my period yet. When it came I had to have my best friend and her mother come over to help me out. This was such a hard time in my life, since I had been so close to my mother. I do not want my daughters to have the same experience. Following surgery I was extremely sore as if I was wearing a coat of armor, stiff, restricting, and heavy. Having drainage tubes hanging on to me was disturbing and made me feel like a patient. I had a hard time with getting out (raising my chest up) of bed and taking showers. My husband helped me through all of this. We have a double-headed shower and he would bathe me. This was a very endearing and close time for us.

(Carolyn S. Olson, diagnosed at age 37)

I was glad to have the mastectomy, as I wanted the cancer gone. I worry about intimate relationships, not feeling sexy. I have a prosthesis and I don't like it. If I were older, I would have the other breast removed. Clothes fit funny. I tend to wear button-up big shirts.

(Cordelia Styles, Quesnel, BC)

I played golf six days after mastectomy. No reconstruction was done immediately because of tumor location. I was in good shape before which aided in recovery. I hated my prosthesis and felt totally unfeminine, so I had prophylactic mastectomy (removing healthy breast) and bilateral reconstruction 18 months later.

(Deb Haggerty, diagnosed at age 51)

I had a mastectomy and immediate reconstruction. This was a good and viable option for me. The plastic surgeon was so helpful and showed me pictures of both implants and TRAM flap reconstruction. We decided this would be the best option for my lifestyle.

(Rebecca Simnor)

The first time, I only had a lumpectomy and radiation. But four years later, I had a recurrence and, at 37 years old, was facing a mastectomy. Devastated, I consulted with five different doctors and they all had the same recommendation. Finally one said, "It is your breast or your life." I caved in. I chose a TRAM flap reconstruction, but the doctors suspected a blood disorder and put an implant instead. The previous radiation to the breast prevented the skin to be stretched enough so I needed a partial prosthesis. Not ideal or sexy but at least I could feel comfortable in baggy clothes at night without the prosthesis, because there was a bump on that side. Seven years later, my implant ruptured. In one day, my reconstructed breast went flat. TRAM option is a more difficult surgery but, if successful, will be permanent. I had the implant removed and replaced two weeks later but had an infection and had to remove it. My options now are to have a TRAM flap, another implant, or have the surgeon just fill the hole and close it up.

(Donna Tremblay, diagnosed in 1992 at age 33, recurrence in 1996)

Take your time with decisions. Reconstruction is a large surgery. Excellent prostheses are available while you decide. Exercise as much and as often as you can.

(Shelagh Coinner)

It's been two years and I will soon have a second mastectomy with bilateral implants because I had two tumors. I have never regretted my decision and would do it again in a heartbeat.

(Yvette, Victoria, BC, diagnosed in 2002 at age 47)

My entire breast was removed. It was very painful. At my age, I didn't have reconstruction. I wear a special bra now with a prosthesis. I've become used to it after all these years.

(Marie, Co. Mayo, Ireland, diagnosed in 1987, recurrence 13 years later)

A year after I was diagnosed, my younger sister had a lump. One of my other sisters suggested genetics and all of my sisters tested positive as well as one of my daughters to date. I then chose to have my healthy breast off and hysterectomy and oophorectomy (the surgical removal of ovaries), all at the same time. I was not prepared to go through the chemo again. The balance problem went away, I did not have to wear the hot prosthesis anymore, and I did not have reconstruction. Two of my sisters did choose to have preventive surgery as well and a reconstruction.

(Marylynn)

After my mastectomy, I was kind of nervous the very first time I saw the result of the operation. I was not shocked, because I had asked in advance how my body would look (scar, nipple or not). I felt my body was out of balance, which still persists today. And I cherish my other breast much more than before. I wore a stick-on prosthesis for one year. Then

I decided to have a reconstruction for the practical part of it and for balance. This reconstruction is well done when I look at myself clothed, but naked, it is not the same. The difference with my real breast is enormous. It feels partially cold, it is not soft (a blown-up balloon), and sometimes it hurts when I have done too many efforts with my arm. I do respect the doctor that did the operation, really, but in comparison to perfect nature the result is rather clumsy.

(Annemie D'haveloose, Belgium, diagnosed in 1999 at age 45)

Life without a breast is different and not easy to accept. I have simply tried to put this loss into perspective. A breast is a small price if you can continue your life. Reconstruction should be carefully considered. Many people say that through reconstruction they have got back their confidence in life as a woman. Others might not be willing to go through this very big and also painful procedure. I think that the most important thing is that your medical system allows you to choose reconstruction if you so decide and also without waiting for years.

(Katariina Rautalahti, Järvenpää, Finland, diagnosed in 1999 at age 41)

My surgical oncologist believed a mastectomy was the best option but, at my insistence, agreed to do a lumpectomy (this decision was approved by a committee of doctors) with radiation therapy and tamoxifen. In May 2000 another mammogram revealed the same cancer had returned at the exact same spot. There was no option but a mastectomy. I had just turned 46 years old and, without hesitation, I decided to have a TRAM flap reconstruction. My surgical oncologist recommended a brilliant female plastic surgeon that could identify with female vanities. After 11 hours in the operating room (each case is different), a day in intensive care, an 11-day stay in the hospital, 3 weeks of daily nursing visits, a home physiotherapist, and feeling at my sickest and weakest, I did not regret my decision for one moment.

(Susan, Brossard, QC)

I don't think I am allowed to have reconstruction because I am at high risk for recurrence. Life without a breast—so what, I have a life!

(Maria Hindmarch)

A radical mastectomy was my choice after I was evaluated by my doctors, because I had very large breasts and the tumor was so deep. After my initial healing, I have used a regular bra with a prosthesis and don't even think about it or ever felt self-conscious except with male nurses.

(Marilyn R. Prasow, Long Beach, CA, diagnosed in 2001 at age 60)

What helped me with recovery was time. This is a hard thing to do. At first you think it is a no-brainer, I'll just have it off. But as time goes by, you miss your boob and begin a mourning period. I hate not having a boob, but I don't want to go through reconstruction right now, it is too much for my young family to handle. I have a total prosthesis and it is heavy. It is hard to believe that our boobs are that heavy.

(Jacqui, Courtenay, BC, diagnosed in 2002 at age 38)

I don't mind having lost the breast as much as being without hair—weird but true. I think it was harder losing the nipple than the breast and I hope that they continue to refine nipple-sparing mastectomy. Luckily my husband has been very supportive, he is warm and affectionate and touches my "boobette" as we call it, though sometimes it hurts a little.

(sams mom)

Accept your new body, embrace it even, and begin moving on. Breasts do not make us who we are. I had a mastectomy without reconstruction. I chose this route because of the young age of my daughter—I did not want to be out of commission any longer than I had to be. Chemo, radiation, and tamoxifen followed. I did have a prophylactic mastectomy and lateral flap reconstruction a year and a half after initial diagnosis.

(Julie Austin, Little Rock, AR, diagnosed in 2000 at age 30)

Lumpectomy didn't seem to change the breast significantly. Ultimately, it didn't matter much since the breast was going to go anyway. I certainly miss my breast... most of the time I am just so glad to still be alive. Sometimes, on rare occasions, and in my most private moments, it really hurts that it is gone. What helped in recovery was to finally have a day where I didn't think of cancer. That took much longer than I thought that it would. In fact, physical recovery took plenty of time, but the surprise for me was how long emotional recovery takes.

(Janel Dolan Jones, Fort Worth, TX)

It helped having my family close by to visit and talk to. I did not have a reconstruction. I was 44 at the time and my husband and I talked it over—he said he did not marry me for my breast but for what I was inside. I wear a prosthesis, but if I had to do it all over again, I would have had both breasts taken at the same time. My life is fine without my breast both emotionally and physically.

(Marianne Svihlik)

I opted for the lumpectomy and radiation treatment. I told the surgeon that I was only 40, and I figured out I had at least 10 years to look good in a great-looking dress! I wish someone had told me that the problems surrounding the lymph node removal would last far longer than any other surgical issues. Now I wear a small pad in my bra to even out my chest; my mother and my husband say they can't tell the difference, but I can.

(Mary Schmidt)

Probably the energy work from my mother-in-law, called jin shin jyutsu (ancient art of harmonizing body, mind, and spirit), was the most important recovery help. Reconstruction begun during mastectomy. The intention was to have an implant after recovering from chemo and radiation. I decided against implant after reading about silicone and saline implants. So I did TRAM reconstruction. Long recovery, not at all what was described to me (two years, not six weeks). Now, three years out, I am finally able to say I'm glad I had it. I am able to wear anything I want and look normal. A breast made from belly fat and muscle is incredibly perfect. Take advantage of the professionals out there who can help with the prosthesis decisions and undergarments, they are really sophisticated now. It's hard to recommend reconstruction, it is a devastating surgery, but as I said I am finally happy I did it. Sad about hip to hip scar across belly, since belly was fine before reconstruction.

(Suzanna Stinnett)

I did not have reconstruction during initial surgery. I still have not made that decision. My reasons for hesitating are the excessive amount of time and number of surgeries involved to replace a breast and ensure both are the same. Surgery and satisfaction are not guaranteed, and there was restriction of some activities (I golf and curl) for the type of reconstruction I selected. I wear a total prosthesis. While healing, I wore loose-fitting garments, then a sports exercise bra and then special bras with the prosthesis. I have accepted the lack of a breast both emotionally and physically, probably more easily than I thought, due to the support of my significant other. Without the muscle in the right side of my chest, my strength and my golf game are not up to par.

(Lorraine)

As soon as I learned I would lose my breast I knew I would have reconstruction. I chose the TRAM flap reconstruction—what a way to get a tummy tuck! The surgeon asked if I wanted to be bigger. I knew that there was no way I wanted an implant in my body so I happily still have my small breasts. I was very sore from my abdomen to my underarm. Then, after the chemo treatments, I had the nipple reconstruction. The surgeon took some skin from my thigh for that. What surprised me was to have no feeling in my left breast.

(Sheryl)

I did not know I would need radiation until weeks after my surgery, otherwise I would not have been given the option of the reconstruction/expander at the time of surgery. I know that I will have scar tissue issues. I loved my pull-on bras for months after surgery. No rubbing or constricting. No underwires! My husband is very supportive of my recovery and my self-image. One breast or two, I am still the same woman he married! He reminds me all the time, so I don't worry about him seeing me differently or finding my body unattractive!

(Lori Hughes, diagnosed at age 35)

Recovery was a breeze, I had to keep telling myself to take it easy, as I was supposed to be an invalid. Ha! I may not have had to do housework thanks to my sister, but I drove my boys all over for their ball games. I haven't decided about reconstruction yet, but if I do get it done, I'd like the other breast taken off and a TRAM flap surgery done. I've watched it twice on TV, and I think that's the way I'd like to go with no synthetic parts to worry about. Life without a breast has been interesting, to say the least. I think my husband has had a difficult time with it, but he denies it, of course. I find using a prosthesis very hot in the summer, especially wearing the expensive one, so I bought a cheapie from a department store, which isn't as heavy and doesn't make me sweat. My attitude about only having one breast is, I'm glad the bad one is gone, so emotionally I haven't grieved for it. There are times when I'd like to wear low-cut tops, but then, I'm 55 years old, not looking for attention from the opposite sex, so why worry about it?

(Cheryl Otting, Elkford, BC, diagnosed in 2002 at age 53)

A lumpectomy and lymph node dissection followed, then a mastectomy and second lymph node dissection, TRAM reconstruction, reduction for other breast, chemo, skin grafts and reconstruction repairs, staph and strep infections, nipple reconstruction, repairs and liposuction, nipple tattooing, and then I stopped! My treatment lasted a year, doing reasonably well, with mild lymphedema and extensive scarring. Think hard about reconstruction. I had no idea of the possible complications. If I'd known ahead what was in store for me, I'd have chosen just a mastectomy. It has been very hard to accept the state my body is in now, and I still have days when I weep about the mess I ended up with. Investigate. There are web sites now with pictures of reconstruction results. Remember that what they are showing is usually the best outcome. It wasn't the mastectomy that bothered me; it was all the complications from reconstruction. After six months I was considering having the reconstructed breast removed. If you decide on a TRAM, be aware that you can't stand up straight for a long time after, because the tummy tuck is the most painful part of it. Plan to spend a lot of time lounging in a C-curve posture, and needing at least three pillows to sleep. Make sure your doctor tells you the warning signs of seroma (swelling caused by accumulation of serum) or infection.

(Judith Quinlan, diagnosed in 2001 at age 52)

I had a total mastectomy of my left breast with implant immediately after. It has been over 20 years so much of the pain and discomfort have been forgotten.

(Roberta R. Nordby, Redmond WA, diagnosed in 1984 at age 29)

Life without a breast is not a problem for me. Full prosthesis is a pain, but life could be worse! I will not consider reconstruction.

(Pat Eveleigh, Vernon, BC, diagnosed in 1995 at age 52)

I was a bra size E and, with the breast gone, I was walking lopsided. Until I finally had a prosthesis, I many times went braless, which didn't exactly look proper. Yet, it did not stop me from going out in public.

(Beverly Vote, Lebanon, MO, diagnosed in 2002 at age 37)

I don't wear a bra. I know it is not the popular choice but I am what I am. I guess I am making lemonade out of lemons, but I decided that I can get by without wearing a bra. I always thought they were so uncomfortable anyway. With no breasts, I guess the biggest thing that I have to be aware of is my posture. I tend to slouch... or lean forward. I guess I am not having too much of an emotional reaction about having lost them. I live my days, tell my story if people want to hear it, and go on. I have a greater reaction when I get afraid that I might get it again and have to go through chemo. Sometimes I wonder if I am a freak because I don't care about my breasts being gone. I think that I fed my babies and they served their purpose, and it was okay to let them go. Two years later, my chest and underarm are numb. I also had a second mastectomy because the symmetry or lack of it bothered me. I have excellent range of movement in my arm. I have had to deal with the lymphedema, which is an ongoing problem and requires constant maintenance.

(Deborah, diagnosed in 2002 at age 46)

I had very large breasts and had always joked that I wish I could just "cut them off"—well I did, but I didn't want to do it this way. I had gone to my doctor for a regular checkup to look into reduction surgery on my breasts. When I had surgery after chemo, they removed my left breast and lymph nodes, but they also did a reduction on my right breast. So I came out of surgery thrilled with my new baby boob, it was so cute.

Reconstruction on my left side would come later after I healed from radiation. If I hadn't had the reduction, I would have been so miserable with that one huge breast. Recovery was much easier being able to go braless and let everything heal. So I never looked at it as losing something because what I gained as a result of this was something I had always wanted.

(Linda Bryngelson, New Brighton, MN)

Surprisingly, I didn't mourn the loss of my breasts. I hurriedly scheduled the mastectomy two weeks later and felt empowered now for the first time in over six weeks.

(Catherine, Pointe Claire, QC , diagnosed in 2001 one month before age 40)

Now I tell people to get a prosthesis because its weight makes you balanced. I didn't for the first while and had to have physiotherapy to get everything back in line. In hindsight, the surgery was the easiest part and yet my most fearful.

(Marylynn)

I am lucky I had no attachment to my breasts. My husband and I put money down on a new house. Our new house kept me from crying many a night. Every time I was having a bad day, I would just let my husband know that we had to go look at the progress of the new house—he understood what was going on, and we would take the drive with the kids. It was no walk in the park after the surgery. I had a two-year-old at home that wanted mommy to pick her up.

(Melinda Flynn)

I was obsessed with looking at breasts wondering if they were real. I am glad the mastectomy was my decision so that I was not left with anger at the medical folks for taking my breast. I have never had reconstruction. I decided it was more than I wanted to put myself through. My husband talked me out of it. By the time my doctor told me it was okay to have reconstruction it was no longer necessary.

(Gloria J. "Mimi" Winer, Point Pleasant, NJ, diagnosed in 1974)

Regaining arm movement

I had trouble with movement of my right arm for quite some time, and I babied the arm. In time I learned I was hurting my situation instead of making it better.

(Beverly Vote, Lebanon, MO, diagnosed in 2002 at age 37)

My surgeon took out 39 of my lymph nodes. They all came out negative, but that result was inconclusive because my surgery occurred after I had chemotherapy—the doctors said that the chemo probably cleaned out the lymph nodes. Because of all the lymph nodes that were removed, my arm mobility was severely limited after the surgery and hurt greatly to move even slightly. I went through a month of physiotherapy and exercises at home to increase my arm mobility to its full range.

(Dikla, North Hollywood, CA)

It is critical to start the exercises right away. My aunt had had breast cancer, and both her arms swelled to double their size. I did not want that to happen to me. It was amazing during recovery how even reaching up for a plate out of the cupboard hurt so much. I wondered if it would ever end, but it did. No one told me it would take so long.

(Carole, Victoria, BC, diagnosed at age 57)

The worst was the lymph node dissection. Sentinel node biopsies weren't yet the norm. I had no idea that I would have a tube or that I wouldn't be able to move my arm without physical therapy. It took a month before I got my range of motion back.

(Leslie, Springfield, VA)

I had a mastectomy and an expander placed under the muscle in the same surgery. Now, ten months post-surgery, I have about 1/4 of the feeling back in my armpit, but the back of the arm is numb. I lie on the floor on my back at least once a day with my hands behind my head to stretch under the arm. After a few minutes, both elbows are touching the floor. It is very important to keep up with stretching to have full range of motion.

(Lori Hughes, diagnosed at age 35)

Probably the best advice I got from my cosmetic surgeon (I had a simultaneous reconstruction) was to use my arm, no heavy lifting, but not to baby it either. Still now, after eight years, there's some stiffness and numbness especially if I'm tired.

(Christine)

For underarm numbness, I went to physio between surgery and radiation. Then after I recovered from radiation, I went twice a week for half an hour. In all, I went 100 times. I now participate in a dragon boating team of breast cancer survivors, paddle on both sides and am almost equal.

(Maria Hindmarch)

I started with eight rounds of chemo to try to reduce the size of the tumor, then I had surgery to remove the left breast. It's hard to explain that numb feeling under my arm and left side. It's gotten a little better than it was, exercises have helped. I got myself some small weights to lift and just kept working at it.

(Linda Bryngelson, New Brighton, MN)

I read everything I could get my hands on and talked to other women going through this mess. My arm was incredibly painful for a long, long time after surgery. I have to admit I wasn't prepared for the level of pain I had for an extended time. I found physical therapy helped loosen up the scar tissue and helped decrease the pain. Now, at six years out, I have permanent numbness but full use of my arm.

(Lee Asbell)

The numbness under my arm is still there four years later, but one gets used to it.

(Joan Fox, Victoria, BC)

I remember my arm being very numb and that I felt like it was sticking to my side. To this day, there are times when it still feels like that. All the nerves haven't regenerated so there are still some areas where I'm numb. And I have a nice attractive dent!

(Leslie, Springfield, VA)

Being in good shape before surgery helped me. I had to be careful about lifting and driving, but I was quickly back to normal. I had to push myself to "walk the wall" to regain my arm mobility.

(S.R., Columbus, OH)

I was told not to use my arm too much, but I did not follow this advise. I started playing tennis after three weeks, slowly, and today I have no problems.

(Karen Lisa Hilsted, Denmark)

After mastectomy and treatments five years ago, the underarm numbness is still a fact, and I don't feel any positive evolution anymore. I will have to live with that. It's sometimes even more than numbness alone. When I have used my arm a lot, there is some kind of tiredness that installs in the whole region. It helps when I do a gentle massage in that area. But, of course, I pay attention not to overburden my arm, and I had six months of physiotherapy after the operation as well as lymph-drainage to regain arm movement.

(Annemie D'haveloose, Belgium, diagnosed in 1999 at age 45)

I went to physical therapy after surgery. It was the best thing I did. The physical therapist pushed the arm further than I ever thought it should go. It really helped me regain my arm movement.

(Johnna Fielder)

The lymph node dissection under the arm was the most painful. As soon as possible, start doing a range of motion exercises to avoid tightening of this area. Walking fingers up the wall in the shower and doing arm rotations are good for this.

(Joni)

My get-well cards not only made me feel better, but they helped me get more motion in my arm. I found it difficult to brush my teeth or comb my hair. So, I taped my cards to the wall. Each day in the hospital, I moved the cards a little higher on the wall until I could raise my arm above my head.

(Gwyn Ramsey)

Lymphedema

Dealing with it, avoiding it

This book is meant to be nonmedical and helpful, not a substitute for professional advice. The opinions of participants are not meant as medical advice to others. Always consult your doctor and medical staff about your specific situation and treatments.

The lymphatic system can be damaged by cancer treatments, including surgery where lymph nodes are removed from under the arm (known as axillary node dissection) and radiation. As a result, the normal accumulation of lymphatic fluid may build up and cause swelling. Known as lymphedema, this distressing side effect can occur immediately postoperatively, or many months or even years later. About 35% of breast cancer survivors are affected by this chronic condition (Lymphedema Association of Quebec).

Many breast cancer patients are never told about lymphedema or how to reduce the risks of getting it. My doctor mentioned it prior to my mastectomy, so I searched for more information, determined to do my part to prevent it if possible. Even now, years later, whenever I become aware of pain after doing something forbidden, like shoveling snow, carrying a heavy load even briefly, or packing boxes for a move, I immediately interrupt whatever I am doing. I elevate and stretch the affected arm and massage it gently until the pain goes away, mindful of seeking medical help if it should get worse or start swelling. I had to learn to be vigilant and serious about being my own advocate. When I had an unrelated surgery some time after cancer, I had to insist that they not use any needles or a blood pressure cuff on the affected arm. The surgeon had dismissed my concerns of lymphedema as irrelevant and the potential risk as impossible.

For up-to-date information, steps to prevention and reducing risks, related booklets and articles, and with links to lymphedema sites, groups, organizations, treatment centers, health care professionals, support groups, newsletters, and conferences, please visit:

www.lymphnet.org
(The National Lymphedema Network, NLN)

www.lymphovenous-canada.ca
(Lymphovenous Canada)

www.infolympho.ca
(Lymphedema Association of Quebec/ Association Québécoise du Lymphoedème)

I am a nurse. I had a lumpectomy of a large tumor with 11 axillary nodes removed. Suddenly, less than four months after surgery, and two months before radiation, I noticed a swelling and puffiness in my left hand. My radio-oncologist immediately referred me for a workup... it was another completely unknown entity and never discussed earlier, lymphedema. The swelling is an accumulation of lymph fluid after the normal drainage system has been compromised by surgery and/or radiation. This was a cruel, gut-wrenching complication, which I found worse than the cancer! At least with cancer, you are given a fixed number of treatments plus medications to ward off the side effects and to hope it won't return; not so with lymphedema. It is a condition requiring daily exercises, manual lymphatic drainage with/without bandaging, and vigilant protection against infection where cellulitis can develop within hours of onset. (Cellulitis is a skin infection of the tissues under the skin, caused by bacteria, with symptoms of tenderness, pain, swelling, redness, fever and chills if infection spreads.) The aim is to prevent irreversible swelling of the limb, known as fibrosis. The psychosocial impact is now being recognized as a major component of the permanent, lifelong condition where one has to wear a graduated compression garment (or orthesis) consisting of a full-length sleeve with hand and finger covering... much like wearing a white cane or announcing a chronic condition like diabetes to the world. I still feel like a freak. The garment itself is a problem—the material, the fit, the daily washing, getting it on with one hand, and keeping it clean (ever tried eating seafood with some finesse using an oversized disposable glove?). On top of this is the exorbitant cost for new garments and the massages. Critically important is protection from sun and insects. I found Sunveil clothing, which gives UVA+B screening. Exercising like walking or Tai Chi is good, also swimming and mild yoga. My advice to everyone, especially with ten or more axillary nodes removed, is to watch for any swelling in the arm or hand, or a sudden infection from an insect bite or injury. No blood pressure monitoring or needle sticks on affected side! This can flare up suddenly up to 40 years later... triggered even by a plane trip (a compression garment is excellent, off the rack). Watch your weight, decrease salt intake, and avoid alcohol if possible. Finally, get an early diagnosis and

AVOID GETTING IT

For the affected arm, no blood pressure cuffs, no blood drawn, no needles. Avoid heavy loads, lifting, and pushing. Avoid carrying heavy handbags or shoulder bags on the affected side. Avoid vigorous, repetitious movements. Avoid tight jewelry, clothes, armbands, and cuffs.

ACTIVITIES

Use a compression sleeve as a precaution when flying or dragon boating. Increase fluid intake when flying. To improve lymph flow, breathing, exercise and stretching help, including walking, swimming, Tai Chi, Chi Gong, and bike riding. Remove your jewelry beforehand.

SPECIALIZED EXERCISES FOR LYMPHEDEMA

Aqua Lymphatic Therapy - The Tidhar Method, Focus on Healing - The Lebed Method (dance & movement), and Remedial Exercises by Dr. Casley-Smith.

SWELLING

If you notice even a slight swelling, massage the arm, keep it up, and monitor closely for changes. See a doctor immediately if swelling gets worse.

DANGER SIGNS

Seek medical attention *immediately* if you experience persistent and increased swelling, limited flexibility, repeated infections, rash, itching, redness, pain, or fever in the affected arm.

PROGNOSIS AND TREATMENT

No cure, but help is available. Best treatment is in early stages. You can reduce swelling and manage lymphedema. Treatments include drainage, diet, massage and therapeutic exercise, skin care, compression garments, and aqua lymphatic therapy. Antibiotics are used for cellulitis (infections of the tissues under the skin). Wear a Lymphedema Alert bracelet or necklace.

assessment ASAP if you have any suspicions, and try to put it into perspective with your whole condition. Don't forget we are so lucky to be alive, no matter a variety of trimmings like daily compression garments.

(MaryAnn, Lachine, QC, diagnosed at age 58)

I don't think there was anything I could have done to avoid it—I think the combination of having so many lymph nodes removed and then radiation put me in a very high risk group for developing it. I did follow their instructions on how to care for my arm, but honestly I was totally surprised when it developed.

(Lorraine Langdon-Hull)

I got it about two years later and have tried everything from the press to the Vodder method of lymphatic massage, physio, sleeve, and on and on. I now do whatever I can manage and then deal with the swelling. Sometimes if I sleep on that side it will drain and I am up in the night. I went to a specialist a few months ago and his letter back to my doctor was "I couldn't tell her much as she has tried everything." The fluid just moves back and forth, sometimes worse, and sometimes the pain is intense.

(Marylynn)

I was shown how to gently massage my hand, arm, chest, and back to help redirect fluids to other lymph nodes that still remained. It worked and aside from a slight swelling under my arm when I overuse it, I don't have a problem with excessive lymphedema.

(Sharon Tilton Urdahl)

I fell a year after mastectomy and hurt my wrist. Lymphedema set in from second finger joints to just above wrist. It's a constant reminder.

(Deb Haggerty, diagnosed at age 51)

I joined "Abreast in a Boat" (dragon boating for breast cancer survivors) and decided to keep active with my arm and not worry about it. I don't feel that activities will cause lymphedema. I purchased a compression sleeve and faithfully wear it when paddling. I also wear it when I fly or when my lymphedema acts up. I feel I have it under control and am lucky I can manage it myself.

(Kathy Reeve, North Vancouver, BC, diagnosed in 2000 at age 32)

I have had trouble with swelling off and on. But I did find the solution that worked for me. I started going to a massage therapist who did Manual Lymph Drainage. We do renos on houses and painting a lot. I usually noticed the swelling after lifting something heavy. It takes a while to get used to the idea that it is not a good idea to lift heavy things, especially hard if you're so used to doing it. I have to be careful lifting grandchildren also.

(Carole, Victoria, BC, diagnosed at age 57)

I have some swelling in my upper left arm. It is not debilitating or painful... just very vexing when wearing short/sleeveless tops.

(Janel Dolan Jones. Forth Worth, TX)

No lymphedema. My partner and I did attend a lecture on the subject, and I perform a massage every day to prevent this from happening.

(Lorraine)

I did my exercises daily for a long, long time. Now, every once in a while I do them (gently pushing the fluid to the other side via massages). I always remember to have blood drawn from the other arm (which isn't easy as chemo ruined my veins). If your veins are ruined, ask them to take blood from a vein in the back of your hand using a "butterfly" device. One day after painfully trying to get blood from the arm, the nurse came up with this idea so now I always tell the nurses to do that.

(Laura, Navarra, Spain, diagnosed in 1998 at age 41)

I developed mild lymphedema about a year after surgery. Before that I had a severe wrist tendinitis—I was practicing a lot of piano for an examination a few months after the chemo ended. I think this was too much too soon. Beware of overuse injuries after chemo and surgery. I use my arms/hands a lot in my work, as a physiotherapist, playing the piano, digging in the garden, chain-sawing the winter's wood, shoveling snow, building projects etc. So far the lymphedema is controlled by wearing a compression sleeve sometimes and pacing myself very strictly.

(Judith Quinlan, diagnosed in 2001 at age 52)

Thankfully, I haven't experienced it. I did get really good education about it during my radiation therapy. I was part of an educational pilot to help prevent it.

(Alicia)

It started about a year later, after doing yard work.

(Bev Parker, Naperville, IL, diagnosed in 1985 at age 40, recurrence in 2001)

Keep your arm on a pillow as much as possible during the healing. Do the exercises. Do not use that arm for blood pressure or having blood drawn from. Do not wear tight clothing—even those tiny gloves one-size-fits-all are too tight to wear. Follow the directions avoiding lifting and carrying things on the affected side. I slept with my arm on a pillow or across my chest and even behind my head.

(Penny)

I wear a medical alert on my arm on the mastectomy side. I can't knit or crochet anymore, since my arm is weak, but I haven't had lymphedema yet.

(Cordelia Styles, Quesnel, BC)

No lymphedema. I wear a compression sleeve when I paddle or fly in an airplane. The only thing that concerned me about the cancer was developing lymphedema because a girlfriend's mother had it and her arm was enormous. I understand that it can come on suddenly after many years.

(Esther Matsubuchi, North Vancouver, BC)

I have not had any problems with lymphedema. I have a pink bracelet that I wear if I go into the hospital saying no blood pressure, needles, etc. in this arm.

(Marianne Svihlik)

Physiotherapy helped me a lot. Sometimes, after a physical effort, I have a kind of pressure in the breast, arm, and back. I massage myself gently, which is giving me relief. Taking blood pressure and drawing blood are always done on my other arm. I still have my port-a-cath for drawing blood.

(Annemie D'haveloose, Belgium)

I experienced some lymphedema during the first year after surgery after I strained my left hand by using a hand ice crusher. The squeezing motion was very difficult, and I really strained. The next morning my fingers were swollen. Fortunately we got right on it with wrapping and physical therapy, and after a couple of months it was under control. I still wear an elastic sleeve on airplanes. I wear a medical ID bracelet: "Lymphedema alert: no needles or blood pressure on this arm." I am scrupulously careful of my left arm now and promptly treat scratches, etc.—this is very important.

(Anonymous)

I am a breast cancer survivor. This experience in itself was devastating, and then three years later to develop lymphedema in my arm was a shock! This chronic condition occurred as a result of lymph node removal and radiation therapy. The physical and mental results were another traumatic experience. I found myself with an invalidity that prevented me from continuing my life in a normal fashion. My arm became extremely swollen, painful, and heavy with reduced motion. I was prevented from doing regular tasks that I had always taken for granted. To my relief, I discovered that I could get help to improve my quality of life, including Complete Decongestive Therapy (C.D.T.), the use of custom-made orthotic support (a therapeutic garment) on the affected limb, and exercises. I started treatments by a specialized C.D.T. therapist and saw a great improvement in my condition.

(Sally Saskin, Montreal, QC)

Chemotherapy

Coping with side effects, hair loss, favorite foods

Wheresoever you go, go with all your heart.
(Confucius)

When the ultrasound did not detect any tumor in my liver, I was eager to start the chemo. The technician said, "Well, I'm not sure I should tell you this, but it's not really that pleasant." I explained I felt it's my only chance. Her advice was, "In that case, the best thing you can do is to go into it with a positive attitude." Chemo was not bad as I expected it to be much worse. Affectionately, I nicknamed the red chemo drug a River of Life, visualizing it running through me and zapping the errant cancer cells trying to hide. I felt the visualization did wonders for my psyche. I watched The Sydney Summer Olympics comfortably in my recliner and imagined myself being those runners, divers, and rowers, with a beautiful, healthy, and strong body, and I felt better and better. I made a long, sectioned cotton bag filled with uncooked rice, sewed it shut, microwaved it for a few minutes and wrapped it around my waist. It helped me more than any pills for backaches, pain, and distress, and it helped me sleep at night. I am still using it years later.

I had good days and bad days. I discovered that being mentally ready to fight is half the battle. I started editing a half-finished book that I was writing, filled with complicated details and calculations. The more I advanced the better I felt. Yet there were also lazy days of "chemo brain" with no work done. My daughter cut my hair short before it fell out—we should have shaved it. When I started losing it by handfuls, I took a shower and saw it falling in the bathtub. Then I saw myself in the mirror and freaked out, looking like a very old woman with a few wisps of hair. I cried and I laughed and then enjoyed showing off my bald head to my family and seeing the expressions on their faces. Losing my hair became an adventure to see how it felt to be bald, otherwise never experienced. It was unexpectedly liberating to shower and sleep without hair. I worked at home so I had the freedom of enjoying being bald. I only wore a wig to go out to make others feel more comfortable. Once I was running in from my car through a horrible storm when my daughter said, "Quick, remove your wig!" So I stood there with icy rain drumming on my bald head and felt totally alive.

Hair loss was not a big problem. I had informed my kids that I would lose my hair. I ordered a beautiful straight-hair, copper-colored wig, completely different from my normal black curly hair. I took it as an experience to be different of how I normally am. It was very amusing going around and seeing friends that would not recognize me.

(Elisa)

Losing my hair caused me to let go of my lifelong obsession and attachment to it. No more curling, coloring, or bad hair days. I wear it as short as I can and love the gray that grew back in. It's my badge of honor and adds to my individuality. Another way to simplify my life.

(Alicia)

Whenever I had chemo I would picture little Pac-Men going in there and gobbling up the cancer globs. When I told my nurse she laughed and said that was a very good visual to have. I don't know how that idea got in my head, but that's how I pictured it. Maybe it came from my doctor telling me how the chemo worked and what it was going to do in my body. I got sick but after changing my nausea medication it got

PORT-A-CATH

If you have weak veins and will need a port-a-cath for chemo and drawing blood, have it installed during mastectomy or lumpectomy to avoid a separate surgery.

STAY HYDRATED

Drink water or other liquids (milkshakes, fruit juices, herbal tea, sliced ginger in cold or hot water, suck on popsicles) before your chemo session so the nurse can find your veins easily, and to flush out the toxins from your body.

AVOID INFECTIONS

Ask you doctor if you should get a flu shot. Avoid all contagious infections during chemo, since your immune system is compromised.

AVERSION

Some have an aversion to water, fruit juice, anything acidic and citric, beef, salty or bitter or spicy foods. Tomatoes and tomato juice appeal to some but not to others.

---

better. I lost my taste for pretty much everything, but soup tasted pretty good as well as toast and vanilla ice cream. I also craved Big Macs which was strange because I never ate those things, but they sure tasted good to me now. But I haven't had one since, can't even look at them. Losing my hair was the most traumatizing thing for me. I didn't look sick till my hair was gone, then you're reminded every time you look in the mirror. Before I lost it I went to get fitted for a wig and, when I wore it, no one could tell the difference.

(Linda Bryngelson, New Brighton, MN)

I didn't experience any adverse side affects from chemo. When I was told I would lose my hair which was almost waist-length, I went to my coworkers and told them I was in cancer treatment and wanted to shave my head as a fundraising effort for cancer research; they donated over $3000.

(Dawn, Victoria, BC)

What helped me a lot to get through chemo was getting pissed off that I had this disease.

(Debbie Peake)

My husband kept on reminding me that all the side effects were a small price to pay.

(Esther Matsubuchi, North Vancouver, BC)

My experience with chemotherapy wasn't very bad. I had heard all these horror stories about fatigue, vomiting, loss of appetite and, to my good fortune, none of those occurred. I even continued to do my usual workout routine. After losing my hair, I preferred wearing baseball caps and hats to a wig. I was now ready to go anywhere lickety split. Take a shower and throw on a hat, how easy is that! It helps to look for the silver linings during your journey. Actually, it is quite a shock watching your hair fall out in clumps down the drain and eventually seeing yourself bald. Being bald for me was a constant reminder everyday that I was a cancer victim.

(Carolyn S. Olson, diagnosed at age 37)

The only complication came after a particularly stressful Board of Education meeting the previous night, and my blood pressure was so high they sent me home. That was a wake-up call, and I decided to resign from the Board to concentrate on my health. I heard that chemo tends to make you gain weight, so I enrolled in a water aerobics class at the local Y as a preventive measure. Now, 7 years later, I'm still doing it.

(Anonymous)

Chemo was the worst experience I've had in my whole life. It totally takes control of your body. I never was nauseated but, after the second cycle, weakness hit me so hard I was in bed for four days. It's so hard to describe. I couldn't stay up but I couldn't sleep. I couldn't read, watch TV or listen to music. My mind raced and I dealt with almost toxic anxiety. Yet I only missed 10 days of work in the 12 weeks of chemo. And I never missed one Friday night of our tradition of Chinese food.

(Alicia)

With chemo, some people have a much rougher time than others. I was one of those people. It made me very ill and my blood counts would

FOOD AND DRINKS

Avoid having an empty stomach; eat small meals and snacks frequently. Everyone is different and the taste and appetite fluctuates. Use common sense and eat a normal, well-balanced and varied diet. Nutritious food is preferable but eat what feels good, especially soft and moist foods, lukewarm or cold. Plastic utensils reduce metallic taste. Try potatoes, spaghetti, noodles, creamy sauces, macaroni and cheese, oatmeal, cream of wheat, bananas, applesauce, scrambled eggs, cheese, burgers, popsicles (make them from organic fruit juice to avoid excessive sugar), dairy products, cottage cheese, frozen yogurt, sorbet, pureed vegetable soups, puddings, vanilla milkshakes, comfort foods, soy or rice milk, fruit smoothies, protein drinks, soft yogurt cheese, pureed baby fruit, yogurt, sour cream, kefir, buttermilk, regular and herbal teas, soups, plain toast, plain angel food cake, vanilla ice cream, rice. Test other drinks if water starts tasting like metal.

**DRY MOUTH, MOUTH
SORES, TEETH**

Drink plenty of water.
Rinse your mouth
frequently with water,
Magic Mouthwash and
moisturizing gels (your
doctor will recommend
what to use, and your
pharmacist will prepare
it for you to have on
hand when chemo
starts). Gargling with
Tea Tree Oil (from
health food store) and
water. Gargling with
a solution of baking
soda and water. If you
don't have mouth sores,
you might be allowed
to use ultra-soft baby
toothbrush; soften
it in hot water. Ask if
Water-Pik (personal oral
cleaning system) is
allowed (regular
toothbrush and dental
floss are forbidden).
Apply moisturizing lip
cream frequently. Suck
on tart lemon candies or
hard mints to produce
more saliva (rinse with
water frequently to avoid
cavities). Avoid or limit
coffee, tea, alcohol,
colas. If possible, see a
dentist before chemo
starts for cleaning your
teeth and fixing any
cavities.

drop so low the nurses would be phoning me at home to see if I was alright. When I was feeling well I ate whatever I wanted. I deserved it. A good wig is a wonderful thing. Not only does it make getting ready to go out very simple and quick, it makes you feel normal. No one looks at you with those sympathetic eyes, making you conscious of your condition. You can spend a day out and almost forget you are sick. I loved just being able to put my hair on and go—it was fabulous.

(Jennifer, diagnosed in 2001 at age 27)

I had all the side effects possible and no medication helped. When I lost my hair, my husband did not like it and told me, "You don't have to look at it!" My daughter was sad at first but later was very proud of her mother—my boys thought it very "cool." Plan your life between the chemo treatments and do this before you start. I got very sad at times but had decided to be "the running, bald chemo-patient." I ran everyday, not fast, but I did it everyday. When I didn't feel like it, my family forced me out, and when I came home I was happy again, and the tiredness chemo gives you was gone for some hours.

(Karen Lisa Hilsted, Denmark)

I was not able to do the fourth treatment due to complications so I was not allowed to participate in the Herceptin clinical trial that I had chosen after much research. My creative solution for dealing with hair loss was to wear hats. This was the worst part of the treatment. Losing my hair for a few weeks would be tolerable but when you are looking at 8 months, it feels like you are carrying a sign "I have cancer!" All my normal routines were affected—I was too sick to even think about cleaning, eating, or washing clothes. My cats were by my side constantly for four months. Without them, I do not know what I would have done. I lost interest in food and lost over 20 pounds.

(Sharron, diagnosed in 2002 at age 62)

My hair was my pride. It was more difficult dealing with the loss of it than the loss of my breast. I bought some really cute hats. I absolutely detest those turban things. I was learning to laugh again. I remember going out on a really windy day without my hat and chuckling at the fact I didn't have to get bent out of shape because my hair might get messed. As sick as the chemo made me, I'm thankful and fortunate that these drugs are available. I gained a lot of weight; chemo made me very ill so every time I felt queasy, I would eat to stop it. I experienced sensitivity to some smells and tastes during and after treatments and even today. I was unable to look at anything red for a very long time. Perfumes and aftershaves nauseatingly smell like fly spray, and garlic, vinegar and olive oil were intolerable. I was just too tired most of the time to do much other than become intimate with the couch. My husband, a wonderful cook, would make anything my heart desired.

(Virginia, diagnosed in 2001 at age 57)

I wanted to live. How did I get through it all? I kept myself busy, very busy. I lived my life as if everyday was my last.

(Melinda Flynn)

NAUSEA

It fluctuates with chemo cycles. Try taking your prescribed antinausea drugs a couple of hours before the chemo session. Food and acupuncture might help. Try Dramamine (Gravol), a few slices of fresh ginger in hot or cold water, gingersnap cookies, candied ginger, peppermint tea, sport drinks, ginger ale. Keep a plastic bag with you in case you must vomit with no rest room nearby.

CONSTIPATION AND DIARRHEA

Test different remedies with your doctor's help. Keep good laxatives on hand to avoid constipation. Moderate exercise and drinking more water might help. Have an extra set of clothing with you in case of accidents if you have gastrointestinal problems.

PAINS AND ACHES

For instant comfort and pain relief, buy a heatbag or make your own version. See page 91.

My hair hurt so much as it fell out. The nurse saw that I was sad and I started to cry, so she told me to go home to get my wig and come back. She cut my hair very short. It was a very emotional moment, but she took all her time to take care of me. I felt relieved yet not quite reassured with the wig (I felt as if I had a dead rat on my head), but I got used to it. After chemo sessions, it took me days before I could eat again. I lost 10 kilos (22 lbs.). Before the operation, I wanted some photographs of my naked body because my body would never be the same anymore with two well-balanced breasts. I also wanted some photographs without my hair. A friend of mine took me to a woman photographer, a real artist, and she took some pictures of me in black and white. They are so beautiful. I didn't show them to many people up till now. But I am very glad that I have a souvenir of that period. What I did most after each chemo was lie down and rest and not move. I had to vomit many, many times, even if I drank just a little water. I had the smell and the taste of the chemical products everywhere. I can still recall that smell now. The best thing to do when I felt sick, was being alone in my little corner. But when I felt better, I wanted to go out, to see my family and my friends, and to enjoy life in the measure that was possible.

(Annemie D'haveloose, Belgium)

I had a pulmonary embolism during the chemo. I felt tired but thought that it was normal. One night I felt like "bubbles" on my chest; it lasted 5 minutes and went away. I mentioned the event to my husband. At the next chemo my doctor asked if I had anything special so I said no, but my husband mentioned that I had complained about the chest pain. To my surprise the doctor became very serious and started asking a bunch of questions. He ordered a set of tests, and the last one showed that I had a double pulmonary embolism. The morale is: always mention your symptoms, always tell your husband or someone about your symptoms, and always bring someone along when you go to your doctor so that he/she can complete your information.

(Elisa)

I bought a real-hair, expensive wig but I rarely wore it. It wiggled, my head was hot, and I thought everyone knew it is a wig. So I became the hat lady. Every food tasted like I was licking the side of a car. Ate jars and jars of crunchy pickles—they seemed to mask the metal mouth.

(Heather Resnick, Thornhill, ON, diagnosed in 1997 at age 43)

I had morning sickness from the treatments, contracted conjunctivitis and lost weight. I felt better if I could talk with my family and friends every day. I have always felt better to say out loud what the voice in my head would keep repeating about the entire cancer ordeal. My taste buds were practically useless. I was eating by memory of how foods should taste to me. I got the food textures, but I needed extreme, strong flavors if I was to taste any food. My food needed to be extremely salty, sour, sweet, or flavored with garlic or onion.

(Kristina, diagnosed in 1995 at age 39)

Chemo was difficult, and I got pretty sick. When I knew my hair was going to fall out, I had a

REST AND WORK

For a few days during each chemo cycle, you are very tired with fatigue deep in your bones, and might feel queasy and lethargic. Rest a lot. Being worn out and chemotherapy don't mix. This is the time to pamper yourself. Outside of those few bad days each cycle you might feel great and run, play tennis, work, live, dance. Some work through chemo and find it helps to distract them.

SLEEP

Sleeping is essential for recovery. Fresh air works better than sleeping pills. For anxiety and stress, try a pleasant walk outdoors and a hot shower before bedtime. Practice deep breathing. Count your blessings. A heatbag calms your tense body (page 91). Try Dramamine (Gravol). Consider professional counseling.

BODY ODOR

Baths or showers with bath oils, gels, or baking soda and sea salt. Non-perfumed body cream.

EXERCISE

Get some exercise to feel better. Take at least a little walk even when you feel dragged out and dead tired. It also helps to prevent weight gain which is a problem for some during chemo and hormonal drugs.

TAKING TIME OUT

Get out at times to feel normal (restaurants, parties, nature walks with friends). Avoid information overload and reading too much if you notice you start believing you have all the side effects you read about.

STRESS RELIEF

Meditate, exercise, turn to your favorite hobby, music, watch movies. Alternative and supplementary treatments: see page 108.

GET HELP, ENJOY

Let friends and family cook, help with childcare, errands, and normal routines. Enjoy what you can, resting, reading, journaling, thinking, doing nothing at all.

party with a bunch of friends, two of whom were hairdressers. They shaved my head, and it helped to give me a little sense of being in control. I did get a wig but didn't like it so I mostly wore scarves. There is much I don't remember, but my husband says I laid on the couch a lot and slept.

(Lorraine Langdon-Hull)

One bit of advice I got was to take a shower every day even if you don't do anything else. I thought that was silly. How could you not do anything except that? But chemo really drains you. Just take it easy, and know when to ask for help. One way I describe it is that sometimes you are so tired, you don't even feel like breathing. It is tough, but it will pass.

(Julie, diagnosed at age 26)

Oh, this was the worst. I bought a good wig and really didn't look sick at all which I think helped. I took all the pills suggested to help nausea, vein pain, dizziness, etc. I think you have to take one day full of pain at a time. And always remember someone out there is suffering more than you. I realized that there truly was such a thing as "chemo brain."

(Joan Fox, Victoria, BC)

Take your prescribed anti-nausea drugs a couple of hours before your chemo. Instead of trying to treat the nausea, I was able to prevent it. If you get mucositis, the lining of your mouth and gums become raw and blistered, which makes it very uncomfortable to eat. You can get a special toothpaste which alleviates it.

(Catherine, Pointe Claire, QC, diagnosed in 2001 at age 39)

Shave your head about two weeks after your first chemo session. You're going to start losing it shortly after that, and your head will hurt. It feels better controlling the time when you lose it rather than just watching it fall out.

(sams mom)

I decided to collect money by shaving my head and giving my hair to the Canadian Cancer Society for Breast Cancer Research. My oldest son who was five thought this was a cool idea. I made an announcement at church and to family and friends as to our intentions, and we started collecting. Three other ladies at church stepped up to the plate and shaved their heads with me and together we collected over $3000. What helped me get through this was my family and church. I pretty much hated every kind of food. I liked tea, and rice in my bouillon. I got sick of water, ginger ale and crackers. I tried cookies made with pot, I ate a lot that night.

(Jacqui, Courtenay, BC, diagnosed in 2002 at age 38)

The steroids to counteract the effects of the chemo made me ravenous, so I ate and just suffered the consequences of gastrointestinal effects afterwards. I gained 20 pounds. The steroids made me hungry, caused insomnia, made my face all puffy and swollen and also made me extremely irritable and nervous. Take your prescription steroids early morning and early afternoon—that might allow you to have a good night's sleep. I could not make any social plans farther than a couple hours in advance, and I always had to be near a bathroom. My drive to the chemo room was an hour in a freeway, an anxiety-ridden trip every time. The chemo also

EMOTIONAL HELP

Meditation and guided imagery during chemo help emotionally and physically. Keep a positive attitude. Visualize your chemo liquid as healing, not only during sessions but many times a day. Take pictures of children, a favorite pillow or blanket, or a heatbag to chemo sessions. You will feel more in control when you know you can find answers to your questions and concerns. Internet message boards, discussion groups, and other survivors will help you emotionally with practical tips, strength, and encouragement to continue. Visual imagery is now offered in some hospitals during chemo.

SUPPORT

Ask someone to go with you to chemo sessions, or take a good book, knitting, or a portable CD player with your favorite music.

VISITS

Even when tired, you might enjoy someone to stop by to distract you.

---

made my concentration fuzzy, and I made more mistakes at work. I had chemo brain at its best. I noticed that the doctors underplayed the side effects from chemo, and the books completely overdid it and scared you half to death. The most realistic expectations I received were from other women going through the same situation.

(Dikla, North Hollywood, CA)

Be sure to drink a lot of water before your chemo. No one told me this before my first session, so the nurse had trouble getting the needle in. Then the next day, the vein in my arm looked dark and bruised. I found out later from another survivor that I should be well hydrated before chemo. I drank about a quart (litre) of water before my next chemo and didn't have any problem with my veins.

(Leslie, Springfield, VA)

I'd feel queasy so I always put something in my stomach the minute I got out of bed (mint tea or a piece of toast). Hair loss didn't bother me. I had long hair, and I had it shaved off. I paid for human-hair wig, because a few days before I had tried synthetic-hair wigs and ended up crying (it looked like they put a helmet on my head). Halfway through my chemo I started using scarves and soft hats. I then slowly built myself up to entering a cafeteria with the hat on, ordering a coffee, and taking the hat off. It was like I wanted to prove to myself that it didn't matter if I had hair or not.

(Laura, Navarra, Spain, diagnosed in 1998 at age 41)

I tolerated chemo but, in reality, I was petrified of its side effects. I rested a lot, even though sleeping was always difficult. I had serious trouble remembering things and extreme difficulty in making decisions about such things as what to wear and what to eat.

(Beverly Vote, Lebanon, MO, diagnosed in 2002 at age 37)

It sucks, but it's totally manageable. Never have an empty stomach. Eat a little bit of something all the time. It really helps. I had my sister shave my head. It allowed us both a good cry and kept me from the ongoing pain of seeing and feeling all my hair fall out.

(Lee Asbell)

I had a port-a-cath put in after the first chemo because I just couldn't stand watching the "red devil" creep its way up my arm. I wish I had had the port put in when I had my mastectomy, but no one suggested it. One thing that was really nice was my friends had a Hat Party for me shortly after chemo began. It was a fun way to deal with a scary process.

(Julie Austin, Little Rock, AR, diagnosed in 2000 at age 30)

My son and I decided to have a shaving party. He shaved off what was left of my hair right before my second round of chemo. I cried for about a minute, then went on with my life. Around Thanksgiving, my best friend called and said she was sending me a ticket to come spend the holidays with her and her family. I began to cry and told her I couldn't come because I didn't have any hair. A few days later I received a box full of hats from her. I ended up flying there a week after my last chemo treatment. I was weak and bald and wondered at times if I had lost my mind, but I had a great time with her.

(Rita, Santa Clarita, CA)

About six recliners were lined up so you could commiserate with the other patients. There was a TV. Nausea medicine was given before each treatment and then I was sent home with pills for the first few days. I found I felt okay until that evening when the nausea set in. Keep that bowl next to the bed. Each person reacts differently. Wearing a wig conjured images of ZsaZsa and Dolly Parton. A wig shop owner was a saint and helped me pick out a wig before I even started chemo and also shaved my head when the time came. She is a breast cancer survivor and carries prostheses and special bras and nighties. She likes you to choose a wig before you lose your hair so she can match it to you.

(Diane Dorman)

Yuck! Yuck! Yuck! I had my first chemotherapy the day before Thanksgiving after receiving assurances from my oncologist that no one gets sick the first time out of the gate. Well, with 26 people in my living room (including a director from one of the top-rated shows in television history), I lay on my bathroom floor becoming familiar with all the makings of a toilet. And to pay the oncologist back for his bad bet, my sisters called him in the middle of his Thanksgiving dinner to call in a prescription. My hair was my focal point and the point of everyone's comments throughout my life, waist-long, luxurious, and beautiful. We cut off my mane to my shoulders, a day later to my neck, then a short-short cut. My husband buzzed my hair off and he himself came home bald that very same day! Everything tasted like metal except for tangerine Altoids, which I ate by the handful—that is, when I didn't have mouth sores.

(Dawn, North Hollywood, CA, diagnosed in 2001 at age 47)

Hair loss was only a trauma at first. When it first came out my follicles hurt. I got the hair clippers and asked my family to help me. It was a ceremony that we will never forget. As for being bald, I felt free. I didn't feel shame or embarrassment about my hair being gone. I wore wigs at restaurants to avoid upsetting others. Scarves were more comfortable for me than wigs, no matter how good they look and feel. Soft woolen caps in the winter were very helpful.

(Janel Dolan Jones, Forth Worth, TX)

Bald is brave! Chemo drug was bad news, pain and side effects, so I was switched to another chemo drug and tolerated it better. Some nails are now deformed so I keep them short and filed-down. I have a wonderful family and worked with a great group of people who loved me unconditionally and accepted me where I was. I had a problem with liquids during the last four treatments. Everything had the texture of a thick gel and that would trigger my gag reflex. Not fun at all!

(psh)

I would go through surgery in a heartbeat over chemo. I somehow can't believe I went through all of this. It just doesn't seem like it happened. I was so scared. Some days I didn't want to get out of bed and I didn't. I survived because of the people God put in my life. I live with my son who was 17 at the time. It is just he and I and our 5-year-old lab, Jake. After the last treatment, I was so dehydrated I had to be hospitalized. My son helped me shave my head and he made me laugh when he said I could get a job on Star Trek. Friends brought me cute hats and scarves. I became quite good at tying scarves around my head. Normal routines? There is nothing normal when you go through cancer and chemo.

(Sheryl)

Chemotherapy was the pits. 6 months of #@^*@! My oncologist tried all sorts of medical combinations that might help, but nothing did. I finally was able to have home health for IV hydration and nausea management. Go to a reputable wig shop before you lose your hair. Take close friends with you. It is a tough day. Laugh often and hard. This is not a time to be by yourself. I had a greater reaction than most people to the chemo, so was literally in bed for almost four days after each treatment and off work for a week. My friends and family knew that I was usually feeling pretty good the week before each treatment and we always did something fun.

(Peggy Scott, Waldorf, MD, diagnosed in 2002 at age 46)

Tough but manageable once you get the idea that you're going to feel like you have the flu... for a solid six months! Emotionally, a strong support network of friends really helped. My coworker left me flowers, balloons, notes, and cards at every milestone throughout the chemo experience.

(Christine)

If I did it again, I would try to avoid reading about the side effects, because you start to believe you have them. I liked popsicles the best. Pizza didn't taste good at all. My advice would be to avoid foods you really enjoy, because you'll develop an aversion to them.

(Johnna Fielder)

I had to go to my journal to remember all the complications and side effects—I guess that means I'm putting it behind me, eh? From a bacterial cold sore on my lip which required antibiotics, to black fingernails, constipation, and hemorrhoids, I found that the hot flashes and night sweats came back with a vengeance. I was so tired and feeling crabby by the fourth treatment, I didn't do any gardening to speak of. I had no energy to go even for a walk. To top it off, the veins in my arm all turned black and hardened, and the nurses kept blowing the veins when they put the IV in. My hair fell out, no problem for me, but I never realized how hot a bald head could get. I only wore a hat—too hot to wear a wig. It was actually pretty funny having a bald head as I'd forget about it and wander around outside or answer the door without a hat on and the people I'd see would be so shocked. I had no energy, but I did manage to continue to volunteer for the Cancer Society as an emergency aid volunteer.

(Cheryl Otting, Elkford, BC, diagnosed in 2002 at age 53)

I got an email from a breast cancer survivor in South Africa, and she warned me not to use an ice bag on my head during chemo to prevent the hair loss. Then I read an article about the same thing with an ice bag possibly creating a safe haven for the cancer cells to return. So I decided it's better to temporarily lose my hair.

(Anonymous)

Chemo was hard. When I was going to have chemo, I bleached my hair blond. That was just a fun thing, something I would never have done before. I got a fever after every treatment. I got burns on my face, hands and feet. I went to work everyday but was not really functional. I was lucky that I had such a great employer.

(Deborah, diagnosed in 2002 at age 46)

I tried lemon, salt, and endless herbal remedies, teas, and diet changes. I must admit that I started smoking again during chemo and this was the only thing that masked that taste—possibly because it covered it with an even worse one! Ha. Marijuana does help with the nausea. My third chemo was on September 11, 2001. Well, that really cheered us all up in the chemo room! Talk about upping the fear factor! Now I wish they'd turned off the TV although, of course, we were all glued to it. I found the nurses and paramedical people were my best source of strength and comfort. Doctors, even the best ones, are just too powerful, carrying control over life and death for you.

(Judith Quinlan, diagnosed in 2001 at age 52)

I was not able to drink orange juice or use salad dressings during chemo, as I found them too acidic. I still don't enjoy orange juice the way I used to. Since having chemo the last time, I have developed sensitivity to certain nuts like walnuts and macadamia—they make my tongue burn and give me sores in my mouth. The day after chemo I would only want to eat a Wendy's chicken sandwich, as for some reason it was the only thing that would sound good. When I felt nauseated, putting my face into my dog's fur and taking a deep breath always made me feel better. There was something so comforting in that. However, smelling his breath was not too pleasant! My husband, Cliff, normally falls asleep the moment his head hits the pillow. However, when I was wired up from the steroid medication given with chemo and couldn't sleep, he would lie in bed and rub my lower back and sing to me; what a sweetheart!

(Joni)

Before my first surgery, my doctor said I would only have to do radiation, and no chemo. After the first surgery, he recommended chemo. And after the second surgery my doctors gave me the choice to do chemo or not. I was so confused. I would change my mind every half-hour—yes, no, yes, no. I got two other opinions from the outside and was recommended to get chemo—why not get more odds on my side? Chemo made me very nauseous and sick. They tried all kinds of anti-nausea drugs, which just made me bounce off the wall. I lost 20 pounds, all my hair, eyebrows and eyelashes. I loved to drink chocolate milkshakes and eat chicken soup and stuffed grape leaves, a Lebanese dish.

(Lorraine Zakaib, Kirkland, QC, diagnosed in 2002 at age 49)

Microwavable heatbag

A heatbag gives immediate pain relief during chemo days, recovery, and beyond. Buy one at a pharmacy or make your own version. Sew a long, narrow bag from strong cotton, leaving one end open (a good size is about the length of your lower leg from knee to heel, and the width from your fingertips to wrist). Fill two-thirds of the bag with uncooked rice or other uncooked grain (but not popcorn!), allowing free movement of the grain, and sew securely shut. Heat the bag in a microwave oven for two or three minutes and drape it around your waist. Massage your aching muscles through the grain to radiate the heat all over for instant comfort.

Radiation

Dealing with side effects, recovery

Nothing is particularly hard if you divide it into small jobs. (Henry Ford)

Despite my mastectomy, radiation was scheduled due to the tumor size and the extensive lymph node involvement. Because I was not mentally prepared to accept it, I found it more difficult than chemo. It took some serious self-talk to change my attitude. I was scared to do it but more scared not to do it, afraid that if the cancer came back and I had not tried everything, I would regret. It got easier after my attitude changed. I only used the cream my radiology nurse recommended. I felt no discomfort and had no burns during the treatments. Only after the treatments ended, as expected, the cumulative effect made my radiated skin red and very painful for several weeks, and then it gradually recovered. The overwhelming fatigue lasted for weeks and weeks after radiation ended. I now know that my operated, radiated site will never feel normal again. Years later, my scar tissue is painful and lumpy, and I still feel occasional stabbing pains shooting through the tight scar adhesions from the mastectomy. At times I feel it is getting worse instead of better. How am I supposed to detect a lump that might be malignant when the entire site is painful and lumpy? It is comforting to go to check-ups and get tests when needed so I can go on with my life with less worry.

I was so overwhelmed that I was in tears. The nurse said, "Take a day off, do something you like, and don't read about breast cancer or think about it for one day." I used to lift the breast to allow the site to aerate. It takes time and you cannot do much, but I would do this as I watched TV. I had a sort of shooting pain as the cells were trying to heal; I was glad to know it was not my heart, as one could be worried. Meditation relaxes you and helps you sleep and therefore promotes healing. Rest when you are tired. Cat naps are great. Walking is good. My dentist said to drink lots of fluids as radiation close to the mouth can cause dryness.

(Penny)

When I was diagnosed a friend gave me the book *Love, Medicine and Miracles* by Bernie Siegel. I found this book to be most helpful in keeping a positive attitude. I was able to do visualization during my radiation treatments and view them as a white light cleaning my body rather than a killing mechanism. I became claustrophobic during the actual treatment and found it increasingly difficult to lie there absolutely still. My solution was to sing out loud. The technician thought I was a bit loony but I didn't care, it helped and soon he was singing with me!

(Sherry Gaffney, diagnosed in 1989 at age 47)

My radiation chamber had a picture of an ocean scene on the ceiling that was backlit to simulate a window looking out over the ocean. I stared at it and imagined pleasant, relaxing thoughts. Sometimes I closed my eyes and imagined other things, like the mountains that

SURVIVOR TIPS

AVOID

Unless approved by your radiation oncologist, avoid all vitamins, supplements, and antioxidants, as they might interfere with the treatment.

TATTOOING OR INK MARKINGS

Some women get tiny permanent tattoos while others get marker lines, depending on surgery. Ask for the difference, recommendation, and availability. Marker lines will disappear gradually. Tattoos can be removed later if they bother you.

INCONVENIENCE

The biggest nuisance is having to go there every day for weeks. Radiation is stressful and tiring. Remember, it is temporary.

SLEEP

Sleep with lots of soft pillows. Arrange them around you for comfort and to support your tender, sore breast.

FATIGUE

Overwhelming physical
and emotional fatigue is
cumulative. Rest several
times a day when your
body needs it. Allow
yourself to heal.

**CREAMS (FOR BURNS, SUN
TAN EFFECT, DRYNESS,
REDNESS, ITCHINESS, PAIN)**

Some creams might
interfere with radiation
or cause allergic
reactions. Use only
natural, water-based
creams without
perfumes, dyes or
alcohol, and only if
recommended
by your radiation
therapist or oncology
nurse. Refrigerating
makes it more soothing.
Start using it when
radiation starts, to
prevent skin breakdown.
Do not put on the cream
just before treatment as
it can cause a skin
reaction and they would
make you wash it off.
Use it after treatments,
also on the exit-burn site
at the back. If you see
blistering, or if redness
spreads outside radiated
area, or if your nipple
and areola become black
and very sore, consult
your doctor immediately.

I enjoy so much. I have a very graphical mind, so I am able to really put myself there and actually hear the sounds associated with such imagery.

(Judi)

I felt very scared, lonely and sorry for myself during my first two radiation treatments. I felt "creepy" being in a dark room on a table with this huge piece of equipment with everyone totally out of the room. But, the technicians were wonderful. They were kind and gentle and each had a great sense of humor. I brought them all a big box of special chocolates.

(Joy McCarthy-Sessing)

I had no trouble except a small burn, about the size of a nickel, like a bit of a sunburn, a bit itchy, and it did disappear shortly.

(Kristina, diagnosed in 1995 at age 39)

The worse thing about radiation is the fatigue. The only way I could deal with it was to sleep for 20 to 30 minutes in the afternoon. Later, I'd sit down and drink water or lie down wherever I could. Fatigue lasted for more than two years with no solution. Eventually, you'll feel your strength return. I swam regularly and went for walks.

(Maria Hindmarch)

I felt my mother's presence with me during my treatments and I found it a comfort to think she was there guiding me. Ironically, my last treatments were on the anniversary of my mother's death from breast cancer 11 years earlier.

(Sharon Tilton Urdahl)

This was the easiest part of my "cut, poison and burn" treatment. I developed a moderate skin burn toward the end of treatments, but it was a piece of cake compared to the chemo.

(Alicia)

Watch out for the exit burn! I was told I may have a burn on my chest, but there was no mention of the burn I would get on my back. So, I was taking excellent care of my breast, moisturizing it twice a day, but I was doing nothing for my back. I ended up with a very itchy shoulder!

(Jennifer, diagnosed in 2001 at age 27)

Radiation was a piece of cake. During my chemo and a year later I did not sleep more than 2-3 hours a night, but during the radiation I got so tired that I could sleep. I had no major complications. I could not run during the radiation but did bodybuilding instead.

(Karen Lisa Hilsted, Denmark)

The most difficult thing was to go to the hospital every single day. That reminds you about your disease. It takes enormous amount of time if you do not live close to your hospital. Major complication for me was skin burns. It helped a lot to put cream on the radiation site every day.

(Katariina Rautalahti, Järvenpää, Finland, diagnosed in 1999 at age 41, recurrence in 2003 at age 45)

It was tolerable. I did get burned, experienced fatigue and found it uncomfortable, but that is what I expected. I had to have radiation on the base of my skull and that was horrible. The can-

COOLING THE RADIATED AREA

After treatment, wet the breast or radiated area with cold water and apply the cream on the wet breast. Bring two cold, wet washcloths inside plastic bags and alternate them to cool down during your drive home. Aerate under a cooling fan with cold compresses. Chamomile tea compresses calm the red skin and help you sleep. Cooling is especially important for large-breasted women as their breasts tend to trap heat underneath or in the axilla area. Go braless at home. Wear loose cotton clothing.

SHAVING

Shaving with blades is not allowed. Ask your doctor if you can use an electric shaver.

SUN EXPOSURE

Avoid sun during radiation treatments. Protect your radiated site from the sun for the rest of your life. Use sunblock liberally (also underarms and on exit-burn site at the back).

BACKACHE ON THE TREATMENT TABLE

A folded towel or a triangular foam pillow under your knees helps.

BATHING

Cornstarch in the bath with a few drops of essential oils relaxes and cleanses (ask if sea salt can be added). Avoid deodorant and perfumed soaps. A mild, natural, organic soap or goat milk soap might be permitted.

PERSPIRATION

Avoid antiperspirants, deodorants, and talcum powder (they contain aluminum, metal, alcohol, and fragrances that interfere with treatments; they are drying and irritating). Use cornstarch or baby powder based on cornstarch to absorb moisture and eliminate body odor. Natural deodorants don't contain an antiperspirant. All-natural crystal rock without aluminum (also in liquid form at health food stores) is a hypoallergenic deodorant (but if it causes a skin reaction, stop using it).

cer spread to the bones in my face, and they were scared it would spread to my ears and eyes so they wanted to do radiation to prevent this. The technicians were wonderful but the treatment was hell! I just had to struggle through and wait for things to get better. They finally did. Through all my treatment I always said I had more good days than bad.
(Kathy Reeve, North Vancouver BC, diagnosed in 2000 at age 32)

My skin did not break but it was red, itchy, and painful. My radiation clinic suggested I apply chamomile tea compresses for instant relief. I seeped the tea in a bowl of boiling water, let it cool a bit, dipped a sheet of gauze in it, squeezed dry and applied over the radiated area several times every night. Then I coated the area with non-perfumed cream. It calmed me and I was able to sleep well. At the last radiation checkup, I got compliments for excellent self-care. Perspiration was my biggest problem. I was desperate until a nurse suggested an all-natural crystal rock; thereafter, everything else was easy. The timer rang to end each treatment the minute I got into a good start in my daydreams.
(Maarit)

Radiation is very lonely. When the time comes and it's you lying on that metal bed with a sheet over it, a cement room, no windows and everyone leaves you, I found it upsetting. I tried to play games in my mind. I burned and it hurt to have even my T-shirt touch me.
(Carole, Victoria, BC, diagnosed at age 57)

I wish someone would have told me that the redness should not go outside the radiated area.

At the end of my treatment I developed an allergic reaction to the cream that I was using on the burn. The redness kept spreading and I kept putting on the lotion. I ended up with a case of severe dermatitis on both breasts. Why didn't I have it checked earlier? I made the mistake many gals do—I planned a vacation to celebrate the end of my treatment. Big mistake. I was away from my doctors when complications set in, and the fatigue was overwhelming.

(Rita, Palos Verdes, CA)

Each week they'd ask if I was tired but I actually felt like the Energizer Bunny, and I had more energy than I had had in months.

(Linda Bryngelson, New Brighton, MN)

Fatigue really got me down. No one adequately explained how taxing it would be. With chemo, you knew you felt bad but it was only a matter of days until you felt better. With radiation the effects were cumulative, and you knew it was going to get worse before it got better. The only time I got depressed during the whole cancer process was the last two weeks of radiation. My skin held up fine, but my psyche didn't.

(Julie Austin, Little Rock, AR, diagnosed in 2000 at age 30)

I wasn't prepared for how I felt getting marked for my treatments. It is quite an experience when you walk out of the office looking like a dry erase board that someone went nuts on with markers.

(Peggy Scott, Waldorf MD, diagnosed in 2002 at age 46)

Going for the first planning session was difficult. Having to hold your arm above your head

PERFUMES

Avoid all perfumed products, including body lotions and creams.

NAUSEA

See chemo chapter for food tips. Your doctor will prescribe nausea medication if needed.

DEHYDRATION AND DRY MOUTH

Drink water and fluids to help flush toxins out of your body. It also helps with fatigue and skin reactions.

POSTTREATMENT DISCOMFORT

Breast tissue might be thicker and darker for many months. Hardening might be temporary or permanent. Some women find mammograms of the operated breast, and even touching it, painful even years later. Scar adhesions can cause stabbing, sharp pains and cramps. After the site has healed, hot showers and gentle massages help. Cold drinks and swimming might make your radiated breast cold, with cramps and pain.

POSTTREATMENT CARE

Cumulative reaction might get gradually worse and last beyond the treatments. Continue pampering the radiated area with your cream. Try Bag Balm for fast relief; warm it between your hands to make it supple (used by farmers, it is now also popular for treating rough, chapped, or dry skin.)

CLOTHING

Loose, soft and cool cotton clothing is the most comfortable. Avoid tight, stiff, synthetic clothing. Use old, dark bras and T-shirts if ink is used to guide the radiation, to avoid damage to clothing. A larger bra accommodates a swollen breast, or go braless while you heal. Layers of cotton tank tops and T-shirts are handy; pin a shoulder pad to the bottom layer if needed after mastectomy. A big shirt over tank top plus a voluminous scarf. For treatments, wear button-down shirts and slip-on shoes so you do not have to tie and untie them to lay on the table.

for an hour and then being poked with tiny blue tattoos all over the place was not my idea of a good time. The radiologist was wonderful and the people at the facility warm and loving. In all truth, it took me 45 minutes to get there, 45 minutes to get home and, I used to joke, 3 minutes on the rack. I handled the radiation with no discomfort or tiredness, but I did burn badly during the "boost." Nothing that gel packs, gauze, and a gallon of aloe didn't help!

(Dawn, North Hollywood, CA, diagnosed in 2001 at age 47)

I went through radiation on my head for the cancer cells found in several locations. I was fitted with a helmet-type device and zapped twice a week for 2 weeks. It was painless. I was told there was a chance that my hair would not return. And, as it worked out, it didn't and the side effect was permanent loss of my hair. After four years, I have a little strip of hair down the back. It seems to be coming in very slowly but it is fine and very thin. However, hats, wigs, and hooded sweatshirts work just fine.

(Roberta R. Nordby, Redmond, WA, diagnosed in 1984 at age 29)

I experienced breast tenderness, feeling of tightness, blistering where the seat belt rubbed, and tiredness that lasted on and off for months.

(Bev Parker, Naperville, IL, diagnosed in 1985 at age 40, recurrence in 2001)

I had no blistering possibly because I took an oral aloe vera solution during the radiation. I was very nervous to begin with, but the technicians soon put me at ease. They were very professional so I relaxed.

(Amy Murphy, diagnosed in 2002 at age 32)

98 • Radiation

Tamoxifen and Aromatase Inhibitors

Hormonal therapy drugs, dealing with side effects

The important thing is somehow to begin. (Henry Moore)

Because my breast cancer was estrogen receptor positive, I started taking tamoxifen. I had virtually no side effects or problems, not even hot flashes especially when I avoided stress and used loose cotton clothing. I was taken off tamoxifen four years later when I developed a massive pulmonary embolism after being immobilized during a hospitalization just weeks earlier. Luckily one of my symptoms, severe shortness of breath, escalated to a point that it finally forced me to call an ambulance, almost too late to save my life. I urge others to be informed and vigilant.

Tamoxifen blocks a tumor's ability to use estrogen. Aromatase inhibitors block formation of estrogen in the body, and they are known as anastrozole (Arimidex), exemestane (Aromasin), and letrozole (Femara).

This book is meant to be nonmedical and helpful, not a substitute for professional advice. The opinions of participants are not meant as medical advice to others. Always consult your doctor and medical staff about your specific situation and treatments.

SURVIVOR TIPS

Pay close attention to your body. Keep notes and report anything out of the ordinary to your oncologist. He/she will know the red flags that might signal rare but serious complications that need immediate medical care. Keep regular gynecological checkups. Get a list of potential complications and side effects from your doctor or pharmacist. Some common side effects are similar to the symptoms of menopause. Avoid soy capsules and isoflavone capsules that might interfere with your treatment. Ask your pharmacist or doctor for their recommendation according to the latest research.

I have had to fiddle with the times I take tamoxifen as I didn't want to be hot-flashing at night to keep me awake. Now I take it in the evening so I get a decent night's sleep, but it does wake me up early. Then I can flash all day if need to.

(Glennis)

I had absolutely no complications of any kind that I was aware of. No side effects.

(Joy McCarthy-Sessing)

I am taking Arimidex. I cannot take tamoxifen, because it raises the risk of blood clots, and I have a genetic marker for blood clotting. Recently my body started producing estrogen again, so I will be having an ovariectomy (also called oophorectomy).

(Dawn, Victoria, BC)

Minor side effect: Hot flashes—wait a minute... it will pass.

(Shelagh Coinner)

My major side effect is joint pain, I feel so old suddenly. And the hot flashes, wow!

(Linda Bryngelson, New Brighton, MN)

One side affect is the cessation of menstruation (boy, that's a tough one) and weight gain.

(Carolyn S. Olson, diagnosed at age 37)

My system began producing more insulin than my body could handle. This resulted in Type II diabetes for which I take a mild medication, not insulin, and with proper diet I have managed to get that under control. Previously I had been diagnosed with osteoarthritis, and the tamoxifen has increased the pain and swelling in my joints. It is frustrating at times, but I keep mobile and that helps. A tamoxifen positive for me has been lowered cholesterol.

(Virginia, diagnosed in 2001 at age 57)

Hot flashes are miserable. I have them sometimes every hour, 24 hours a day, worse at night. I can only suggest natural fabrics, layers, portable fans and any kind of stress reduction activities you can find. I have had two menstrual periods since my 2nd chemotherapy and my family MD makes sure I have endometrial biopsies once a year.

(Alicia)

Not all tamoxifens are exactly the same. Once my pharmacist could not find me my usual generic tamoxifen and I started experiencing such huge hot flashes that they came out of my ears! I went to see the pharmacist and she said that it was impossible because the recipe was just the same. I insisted on having my old generic brand back and when I got it, everything was fine. I mentioned this to other women with the same symptoms and sometimes they realize that their generic tamoxifen was changed as well.

(Elisa)

Tamoxifen caused weight gain. I have decided it is better to be alive and chunky than skinny and dead.

(Jennifer, diagnosed in 2001 at age 27)

I have a lot of hot flashes but, as one of my friends said, "Enjoy the heat!" When I was in

VAGINAL DRYNESS AND ITCHING

Drink lots of water. Avoid douches and perfumed soaps and toilet paper. Keep your vaginal area very clean. Shower head set on massage mode gives instant relief. Wear panties with cotton crotch. Remove panties when sleeping. For intimate relations and comfort, try over-the-counter water lubricants and moisturizer gels like KY Jelly or Replens. Your gynecologist will prescribe other products if needed.

LEG CRAMPS

Eat fruit and veggies high in potassium such as bananas, dried fruit, and tomatoes, and drink fruit juices. Drink lots of water. Try a few slices of fresh ginger in water for hot or cold tea. Soak your feet in hot water. Exercise. Massage your legs. Stretch your legs, elevate and rotate ankles, stretch calves by pressing your feet against a wall.

my tent in Argentina on a mountain climbing expedition, and my feet were frozen, I waited for my hot flashes and enjoyed them. But, as my friends say, I am not normal. (An international team of seven women with breast cancer past climbed Mount Aconcagua in Chili-Argentina in 2004; please see http://www.BeyondTheWhiteGuard.org)

(Karen Lisa Hilsted, Denmark)

After a lot of research I decided that I wanted to take Arimidex instead. Because of the risk of bone density loss, I am also on Fosamax. I have had no side effects or problems with either pill.

(Sharron, diagnosed in 2002 at age 62)

I take Nolvadex for the fifth and last year. Since the operation, I am menopausal. This is something that is difficult to accept. There is a step in your life missing. From being a woman with regular menses you become a woman without any. Never more. No transition period. Strange. I'm sometimes very embarrassed with the flushes I have. They come unexpectedly, mostly in situations that you really don't want them to appear (a face-to-face discussion, for instance). And I know that it is very, very visible. I'm as red as a lobster!

(Annemie D'haveloose, Belgium)

I refused tamoxifen. I may regret it. But I'd had enough of medicine, and reading lots of studies didn't convince me it was any safer than the risks of recurrence I already faced.

(Judith Quinlan, diagnosed in 2001 at age 52)

I took tamoxifen for over eleven years and was told in 1997 that I should have taken it only five years. The doctors believe that this length of time contributed to my cervical cancer in 1990. Today I am happy to be a survivor.

(Gwyn Ramsey)

Possibly it is making me moodier, but I can't tell for sure if it is the tamoxifen or just the moving on after a year of cancer treatment that is causing my emotional seesaw. No hot flashes.

(Dikla, North Hollywood, CA)

No adverse side effects. I have gained weight, but I'm also four years older and think it comes sometimes with the territory.

(Rebecca Simnor)

Hot flashes were a real pain, but they have mitigated since going off tamoxifen after five years. I also experienced some shortness of breath, a less common side effect. Tamoxifen is a known bone-builder, which was important in my case because I have a family history of osteoporosis. That was why I had taken estrogen for all those years. I have lost bone density even though I drink lots of milk and have plenty of calcium. So now I take a bone-builder once a week and increased calcium.

(Anonymous)

I took tamoxifen for seven months and had all kinds of complications. I finally asked my GP to send me to the Cancer Agency for a second opinion and went off it.

(Marylynn)

I have been on it since four and a half years, and I still have heat/cold intolerance. It does give me an increased appetite. I have no solutions but to go off it which I certainly will not do, since it is keeping me alive.

(Maria Hindmarch)

I took tamoxifen and then Femara for about a year. Then the cancer stopped reacting to these estrogen blockers and found another source. At that time my oncologist took me off these drugs. I don't feel I experienced side effects with these drugs. I underwent a full hysterectomy in May 2001 as the cancer had spread to my uterus, cervix, and ovaries. Estrogen blocking was not needed after this surgery.

(Kathy Reeve, North Vancouver BC, diagnosed in 2000 at age 32)

I took tamoxifen for 15 months and didn't like what it was doing to me. Under the supervision of the new oncologist I discontinued it.

(psh)

I'm on tamoxifen now after the recurrence three years ago. I have occasional leg cramps, but otherwise no problems.

(Bev Parker, Naperville, IL, diagnosed in 1985 at age 40, recurrence in 2001)

I took Zoladex for 2 years and tamoxifen for 3.5 years. The hardest and worst part was vaginal dryness and decreased sex drive especially since I was a newlywed. The worst thing you can do is stop having intercourse, because when you are that dry you "shrink" and then intercourse is painful. It puts you in a vicious circle that leads you to not having sex. I wish someone had told me that ahead of time. Still difficult for me physically and emotionally. You and your body get used to not having intercourse, and it's tough to start again.

(Julie, diagnosed at age 26)

Tamoxifen may save my life, but the drug side effects suck. I'm 44 years old, and for the last 4 years I've suffered the effects of menopause without actually going through it. Night sweats, hot flashes, emotional instability. And to think that a tiny little pill is making me feel like an alien. There has to be a better alternative for premenopausal women.

(Mary Schmidt)

Since four years. No major side effects or complications. Makes you very hungry, must fill up on fruits and veggies. I suspect that it is responsible for my loss of libido, but will not know until I finish.

(Anonymous)

After being on tamoxifen a year, I had a routine eye exam and had developed cataracts. The doctor consulted her medical books and found out that cataracts can be a side effect of tamoxifen.

(Leslie, Springfield, VA)

Make sure you tell your oncologist exactly how you feel, since they don't know unless we tell them.

(Peggy Scott, Waldorf, MD, diagnosed in 2002 at age 46)

I took tamoxifen unhappily. Hot flashes and feeling like I was going crazy inside my own skin didn't sit well with me. Extreme self-care and wellness is my therapy.

(Janel Dolan Jones, Forth Worth, TX)

Hot flashes are a side effect, but I feel like it's worth it to be alive.

(Johnna Fielder)

I was prescribed an antidepressant that some use for hot flashes. It doesn't help so it's just sweater on, sweater off! Also, it causes constipation for me, but it's something I have to live with.

(Joan Fox, Victoria, BC)

The only side effect I experienced for the first six months was hot flashes. My friend called it my own personal summer. They didn't bother me because I am always cold anyway.

(Sheryl)

I was 46 when I was diagnosed and had already begun menopause with hot flashes. I don't really know how much or how little the tamoxifen contributed to them. When I got a really bad hot flash I would either go outside or stick my head in the freezer depending on the time of year.

(Sherry Gaffney, diagnosed in 1989 at age 47)

I hate it as much as the chemo treatments. It gives me wicked hot flashes and night sweats and there's many a day when I'm cranky. These hot flashes are a lot worse than the menopausal ones I went through. I also get leg and foot cramps, but I find that if I eat bananas most days, I don't get them. Due to the tamoxifen stopping the production of estrogen in my body, I have atrophic vaginitis and intercourse is very painful. Definitely a complication, I'd say. The flashes catch you when you're either in a meeting, in the car with the heat turned up and it's minus 40°C outside, and the passengers don't understand that I'm burning inside while they aren't. Great conversation piece! A couple of ladies at my support group don't have the flashes (Chinooks we call them), although one had had them for about 4-6 months, then nothing. Lucky her.

(Cheryl Otting, Elkford, BC, diagnosed in 2002 at age 52)

Unfortunately, Arimidex gave me joint and bone pain so I returned to tamoxifen. Hot flashes, mood swings, and body fatigue. But I have not found an alternative.

(Lorraine Zakaib, Kirkland, QC, diagnosed in 2002 at age 49)

No complications. Side effects: initially extreme sweats—at night, in the middle of the day, every 45 minutes or so. Also, weight gain and a strange sense of euphoria—situations at work that ordinarily would have had me being upset about, I found myself laughing over especially if my boss was fussing at me for something. I am taking prescription drug for hot flashes, and it helps a lot.

(Debbie Peake)

I couldn't take tamoxifen because I have a history of deep vein thrombosis. The doctor prescribed Femara instead. The side effects include depression and hot flashes, but I am just relieved I can take something to help prevent recurrence.

(Marilyn R. Prasow, Long Beach, CA, diagnosed in 2001 ate age 60)

I did not have to take tamoxifen. If I wanted to I could have, but it was not a recommendation for my regime. If someone wants to do everything possible and would feel better psychologically doing everything available you could. We really can make our own choices. I felt personally for me the risks outweighed the benefits.

(Penny)

Antidepressants help with the flashes and my ability to function and cope with daily life.

(Deborah, diagnosed IN 2002 at age 46)

Five years of tamoxifen. I can't remember any side effects.

(Esther Matsubuchi, North Vancouver, B.C.)

Complementary and Alternative Treatments

What might help, what might harm

First, do no harm. (Hippocrates, 450 - 355 B.C.)

Used in conjunction with standard medical treatments and with your doctor's approval, some nonmedical complementary treatments might help relieve pain and emotional distress. Such complementary treatments include visualization, guided imagery, muscle relaxation, deep breathing exercises, meditation, self-hypnosis, biofeedback, massage, Reiki, osteopathic treatments, acupuncture, yoga, and Tai Chi. Many find help in journaling, spirituality, distraction with pleasurable activities, laughter, nature, walking, exercise, learning to use the mind-body connection, and even holding an amethyst or crystal to focus your thoughts on healing. The presence of water has a therapeutic, calming effect. Eat a well-balanced, healthy diet to meet your nutritional needs. Some patients may need counseling, mild antidepressants, or sleeping pills to get through treatments.

Cancer makes us feel vulnerable and confused, anxious to do something and willing to try almost anything out of the ordinary, including alternative methods instead of standard treatments. But beware and don't take any herbal medicines, vitamins, or supplements without your doctor's approval. They are not always adequately studied, and they might react adversely with the treatments, posing serious risks to the patient. Don't use unregulated or illegal supplements or megadoses of vitamins with wild and sensational promises. Don't self-medicate or use chatroom tips to change your treatments without your doctor's knowledge. Get reliable information about the latest findings. Don't be intimidated by anyone, including your well-meaning friends, to play games with your health. Don't take unnecessary risks.

A friend suggested alternative treatments and bizarre products to heal my cancer instead of using standard medical treatments. She was annoyed when I refused. Between chemo sessions, I enjoyed osteopathic treatments, non-invasive and pleasant. To calm down my turbulent thoughts and fear, I visualized, meditated, and practiced deep breathing, confident that such things cannot possibly hurt me.

I believe that each person must decide for herself. *Choices in Healing* by Michael Lerner provides good, reliable information. Beware of inflated promises.

(Shelagh Coinner)

I had a lot of healing parties with friends and even put a healing altar next to my bed. It had on it everything from every religion you could possibly imagine. I kept the altar in place during my entire chemotherapy. I was advised not to add anything to my body that is not naturally found there (vitamins and supplements in a larger dosage has never been tested with chemotherapy), and therefore my oncologist was not comfortable with my taking homeopathic remedies.

(Dawn, North Hollywood, CA, diagnosed in 2001 at age 47)

Many people sent me articles and called me about alternative therapies. I read books and found some on my own. I experimented with Tai Chi, visualization and meditation techniques. My visualization attempts during radiation turned into cartoons, every time. I just kept visualizing this fluffy cloud as the healthy cells and this really ditsy black cloud as the cancer cells. It was kind of weird. Meditation helped me considerably. I tried many different types and with tapes, but the best was the breathing meditation, where you focus on your breathing and count your breaths. I felt better than I had felt in years with just 10 minutes in the morning and 10 minutes later in the day. It gave me energy and kept me calm and peaceful.

(Donna Tremblay, diagnosed in 1992 at age 33, recurrence in 1996))

Counseling is a very good idea.

(Jennifer, diagnosed in 2001 at age 27)

I tried naturopathy, Traditional Chinese Medicine, and have researched and taken supplements and antioxidants. My regime is brisk walking daily and a high fiber diet.

(Yvette, Victoria, BC, diagnosed in 2002 at age 47)

I went to a naturopath prior to lymph node surgery, took lotions and potions and pills. My doctors were aware that I was seeing naturopath and didn't necessarily approve. Going to the gym really helped me. My GP knew what supplements could affect my conventional therapy and we stayed clear of them.

(Heather Resnick, Thornhill, ON, diagnosed in 1997 at age 43)

I went to a herb doctor. He gave me a treatment as a kind of counterbalance against all the chemical products that went around in my body. I think it did me real good. I took some vitamins and supplement. I told my chemotherapist about it, but she was not very enthusiastic and said, "I hope these products are not toxic."

(Annemie D'haveloose, Belgium)

I was going to physiotherapy several times a week. After the axilla dissection, I had developed a frozen shoulder and was in absolute agony most of the time. My therapist, a young Asian girl, suggested I try acupuncture. No thanks, I have had enough of needles. But as time progressed and the frozen shoulder didn't improve, I decided to give the acupuncture a try. Lo and behold, after only a few treatments I was able to raise my arm above my shoulder. With diligent exercising and continued therapy, I am now able to do almost anything. I exercise daily using half a broomstick to reach as far as I can above my head. Simple exercises have kept me mobile. Later I began Tai Chi. What a wonderful experience! I am becoming a believer in the ancient Chinese ways. Tai Chi for me has been a lifeline to looking and feeling better.

(Virginia, diagnosed in 2001 at age 57)

I found being open to all the healing options offered to me gave me a sense of having some control in my life, at a time when I needed it most. Keeping focused on healing rather than dying gave me more power over my choice to live. I walked daily because the nervous tension had built up so much that I had to release it physically. I tried a variety of healing methods, from going to a "Peyote healing ceremony," relaxation tapes and meditation and First Nations Sweat Lodges. The nights were the worst, sleeping was a problem for me. There were no distractions when the rest of the world was sleeping and I couldn't seem to shut my "dark" thoughts off at bedtime so I finally agreed to take a sleeping pill. I had read that the body heals while we sleep. During my radiation treatments I took a natural product called Valerian as a relaxant. I had chosen to take a spiritual and naturopathic approach and combine it with conventional medicine to try and heal my body, soul, and spirit. I went to a naturopathic doctor and, under his care, began to feel stronger physically and mentally. I joined relaxation groups and took an art therapy session.

(Sharon Tilton Urdahl)

When I first came home, I was into the healthy lifestyle mode and probably drove my family crazy with healthy eating, over-the-top paranoia, and finally I did quieten it down a bit. I try to be careful although I don't think my diet caused breast cancer. I do yoga, am back at the gym and I dragon boat, which is wonderful. I try to lead a less stressful life, and I definitely look at life differently.

(Rebecca Simnor)

During chemotherapy and radiation, I used complementary therapies, including acupuncture and supplements. The nutritionist I went to works at the same hospital I was treated at and is a physician himself. He looked over my medical file and created a specialized supplement and vitamin list for me to take to boost my strength and immune system, to alleviate side effects as well as making sure none of the supplements interfered with any of the treatments.

(Dikla, North Hollywood, CA)

I practice biofeedback (a treatment technique in which people are trained to improve their health by using signals from their own bodies) for a disability of many years which also helps me relax. I try to walk and take vitamins.

(L.C.)

The doctors didn't recommend any complementary or alternative treatments at all. However, from a friend, I learned about Essiac tea and this really helped how I felt. I wish that nutritional therapy was part of the healing program for patients today. I am a big believer in alternative and complementary procedures. I have learned about the oils for healing, hands on healing, nutrition, emotional release, and more.

(Beverly Vote, Lebanon, MO, diagnosed in 2002 at age 37)

I feel that cancer treatment is a big puzzle with many pieces. Traditional medicine, complementary/alternative therapies, and spirituality are all needed to help deal with cancer. Each serves a purpose. I have used massage therapy, acupuncture, a homeopathic doctor, a naturopath, and a nutritionist. I have attended relaxation classes, cancer retreats, support groups, yoga classes, and Tai Chi. I also use relaxation and guided imagery. My oncologist has been very supportive of these alternatives. I have not been using any naturopathic drugs since I have been in active chemo treatment.

(Kathy Reeve, North Vancouver, BC, diagnosed in 2000 at age 32)

I did relaxation and visualization during my chemo and then listened to a special tape I had when I would go to bed. My surgeon was very happy knowing I was using the tapes. He also suggested keeping a journal.

(Marianne Svihlik)

I asked my oncologist at the Cancer Clinic about natural estrogens in soy products because some tumors are caused by excess estrogen. She said not to drink 8 cups of soymilk a day and to have tofu in moderation. Vitamin C during radiation can interfere with the treatment.

(Penny)

Tried hypnosis but it didn't help. Took some vitamins during treatment, and told my doctor. High doses of antioxidants may interfere with the radiation or chemo. After treatment, I started taking a lot of stuff to boost my immune system, which had been devastated. My present oncologist was really impressed with my bloodwork and said, "I don't know what you're doing, but whatever it is, keep on doing it!" I told her that I eat a lot of fruits and veggies, and work out every day, but didn't mention the supplements. Many doctors are prejudiced against herbs, and I was afraid that she might say that it had interfered with the tests.

(Anonymous)

One of the most helpful things I did was call my friend who is a psychic healer. She used guided imagery and made a tape of this so I could use it at home. Trying to do this on my own was difficult because my mind was exploding with all the info and emotions, and I couldn't quiet myself. As a lifeline when I started to have negative thoughts, Susan had me memorize six positive aspects of my situation. I also journaled and wrote poetry. The writing process was very healing for me.

(Diane Dorman)

So, did I mention that the tamoxifen is horrible? I started taking black cohosh. None of my doctors could tell me if this was a good thing or a bad thing. None would recommend it and none would tell me to stop. Does it work? Who cares; when I'm on it I seem to have fewer hot flashes and night sweats. If it's a placebo effect, bring it on!

(Mary Schmidt)

I never bothered with alternative treatments although Lord knows everyone tries to offer you one. Psychologically, if I ever had a sad moment, I'd turn on music from the 60s and dance in the house alone, and it really helped. Other times, I'd get in the bathtub and cry my eyes out. Once that was done, I'd get dressed and go out and treat myself to a coffee.

(Laura, Navarra, Spain, diagnosed in 1998 at age 41)

I saw a chiropractor and massage therapist during my treatments. I truly feel these things increased my energy level as well as my mental state. I attribute my relative ease with chemo to incorporating these treatments into my overall cancer plan.

(Julie Austin, Little Rock, AR, diagnosed in 2000 at age 30)

Now that I am medication-free, I am looking into these therapies. A Chinese friend of mine has me drinking green tea everyday. And don't forget... laughter is always the best medicine!

(Julie, diagnosed at age 26)

I've always been the type to take vitamins and supplements, but my oncologist warned me against all of them while I was on chemo. Since my tumor was estrogen receptor positive, I also avoid soy or any type of phytoestrogen. A lot of the low-carb foods contain soy so we need to be aware of this before using these products. Nothing has helped with hot flashes. I know some women have success with antidepressants and blood pressure medications, but nothing has worked for me. I'm ready to try acupuncture! Maybe that would help.

(Leslie)

My sister-in-law sent me vitamins and supplements, and I believe that is what helped me to heal so quickly. I returned to work in four weeks.

(Sheryl)

My medical oncologist's advice about vitamins was, "Don't take even Vitamin C without telling me." I do not take any alternative treatments but I do attend a Healing Circle every week where we do a "Reiki/healing touch hands" on for each person, lasting around five minutes. My Healing Circle is instrumental to my recovery.

(Maria Hindmarch)

I did not participate in any alternative treatments before, during or after my breast surgery. Many of my friends are on hormone replacement therapy, which, of course, I cannot do. They don't know how I can stand it without taking HRT or something. My thinking is that anything, even the so-called natural treatments such as soy and black cohosh and other such remedies are not proven or even regulated, so who knows what they can do, especially in conjunction with some other prescription or over-the-counter drugs.

(Joy McCarthy-Sessing)

I think that alternative treatments can be dangerous if they replace the medical treatment. They may also give you false hope and loss of money. I think that right nutrition is very important. Your diet should be balanced to prevent cancer and also to recover from cancer.

(Katariina Rautalahti, Järvenpää, Finland, diagnosed in 1999 at age 41)

Saw a naturopath, but wasn't impressed. Too expensive, too weird, and she injected my scars with some naturopathic remedy without first asking me. Had a Healing Touch treatment and didn't really get anything out of it. Had another several months later and started crying uncontrollably, then felt lighter and freer than I had in months. Had an auric healing a year after treatment and felt a surge of energy going through my arm and breast. I felt great after, as some of the numbness went away immediately, and my arm pain was gone for hours after. I never consulted my doctor about any of these, but I'm sure he'd be fine about them. I lost a lot of weight on chemo, because I just couldn't eat. I believe now that my body knew what it was doing and semi-starvation was what it needed to fight the cancer. Maybe I'm just fooling myself, but I tend now to not try to "control" my body so much and pay more attention to what it asks of me.

(Judith Quinlan, diagnosed in 2001 at age 52)

I investigated and used lots of complementary methods. I was really looking for whatever would increase my odds of survival and ease the difficulty of my experience. I used meditation and guided imagery religiously, I exercised, tried out Yoga and Tai Chi, attended a Wellness Center support group, journaled extensively, received Healing Touch and massage, and continued seeing my natural health chiropractor. I did take some natural supplements but talked it over with my doctor.

(Lorraine Langdon-Hull)

Meditation, yoga, and journaling. Walking, resting, reading great books. Laughing with friends or funny movies. Not only will it boost your immune system by creating peace of mind and contentment, but it adds quality to your life no matter how long you live. Doctors don't know nearly enough about vitamins and alternative treatments. I have had to seek out everything by myself... even good doctors that are supportive, in general, don't know anything about them.

(Janel Dolan Jones, Fort Worth, TX)

I do a lot of visualization. I feel it is an activator of the immune system.

(Anonymous)

I took baking soda and sea salt baths (a pound of each in a tub of hot water, soak for 20 minutes), at the end of each week to release the radiation. I found it relaxing and cleansing, and sometimes I added a few drops of essential oils, such as frankincense, to the bath. I used pure aloe on my breast. I make my own deodorant with pure, natural ingredients that don't clog the pores. I juiced and it served me very well. Some felt it's too much work but to me, it's live or die. There is no one magic bullet. There are many steps to health, and they all work together. Faith played a huge part in my healing.

(Judi)

I went to get my intestines cleaned but my oncologist scolded me afterwards.

(Maarit)

I see a massage therapist on a regular basis and that is all I really needed.

(Cindy, Cedarburg, WI, diagnosed at age 41)

I avoided all the vitamins and herbs to lessen the risk they would interfere with treatments. I did attend deep relaxation sessions and one-on-one counseling. I also learned to perform therapeutic touch and took aikido classes.

(Dawn, Victoria, BC)

Multiple vitamin... that's all. Herbal tea for nausea.

(Christine)

Fear of Recurrence

Getting through fear, facing a new battle

It takes too much time, being afraid. (Pierre E. Trudeau)

Life is fragile, but we are surprisingly strong when we must be. Each checkup is frightening. Each anniversary is a victory. Each day is a gift. For the first year, I felt that if I didn't watch it all the time, the cancer would sneak back. I finally convinced myself that whether the cancer does come back or not, either way I would be foolish to waste perfectly good time waiting and being afraid, and I decided to feel well and cancer-free until proven otherwise. It works wonders most of the time. I have been through fear and panic several times, in the beginning more, then less, always sure the cancer is back. To get through dark moments, I need to voice the reality of my fear, to accept it, to honor it, and to release it to feel hope again. I am grateful that my family listens to me and comforts me, and that my doctors take my concerns seriously and run tests if needed. Peace of mind always energizes and renews me. I was happy to learn that while breast cancer can recur at any time, the danger of recurrence diminishes with each passing year. I still worry that I might miss the signs of recurrence, but I think about it only occasionally. I notice the cancer's shadow less now that it has moved behind me, and I see light ahead again. Acknowledge the fear. Get acquainted with it, tame it, shrink it, and dance with it. That's how the title for this book came to me while I was dancing alone to the tune of "How fragile we are" by Sting.

Doubts are more cruel than the worst of truths. (Molière)

I am fours years out and still worry whenever anything is not "right." Cancer survivors deal with this phenomenon all our lives. A simple ache is never a simple ache again.

(Julie Austin, Little Rock, AR, diagnosed in 2000 at age 30)

I am totally frightened of recurrence, but I do remember my medical-oncologist saying, "The longer you can go between now and recurrence, the better your chances are." Breast self-examination and mammograms may be helpful for early detection in many cases. With inflammatory breast cancer, if your skin goes red and feels hot, make sure that a doctor hears you. It waxes and wanes. You and your doctor won't be able to see it all the time. Insist on a biopsy.

(Maria Hindmarch)

I read about breast cancer, but I will not let it consume my life. Yes, I feel very discouraged to hear someone has died from breast cancer or any other type of cancer for that matter.

(Joy McCarthy-Sessing)

I'm constantly torn between wanting to do BSE every day and never wanting to do them again. I still do them monthly. I've tried to maintain a good weight, do yoga and some aerobic exercise. I still try to follow a low-fat, no-red-meat diet. It's very hard to hear about other people with any kind of cancer. I think BSE is extremely important. My mammogram did not detect the lump. We should take advantage of every means of early detection.

(Alicia)

I was 16 years cancer free. I am not sure why I had a recurrence but keep going back to the stress factor. X-ray of chest found a tumor in the lung after I had a long term cold with a cough. Biopsy revealed recurrence and several other tests found traces in the brain, neck, bones and back. I found a doctor who offered positive

SURVIVOR TIPS

Ask your doctor what symptoms need urgent attention. Report anything unusual to your doctor (persistent new pain, any change in your breast, redness or rash, new lumps, possible infections, discharge from the nipple, dimpling of breast, bone pain, loss of appetite, unexplained weight loss, headaches, dizziness). Keep notes so you won't forget by the time you see your doctor.

When you are afraid, write it down, list your reasons for fear and evaluate them.

We all have aches and pains, often from overuse or underuse of muscles, and most of them disappear overnight or in a few days. It will get better gradually. You will soon get more comfortable waiting for a week or two to decide if you need to see a doctor. Always follow your intuition; if you feel something is wrong, see your doctor.

options and diagnosis for me. I have a very positive attitude and a child (age 11) who makes my determination to be a survivor even greater. I will not allow this disease to beat me! I believe in good medical maintenance, early detection, and a good relationship with your doctor.

(Roberta R. Nordby, Redmond, WA, diagnosed in 1984 at age 29)

Recurrence is not an automatic death sentence. Miracles happen all the time. I am a cancer warrior. I have all the tests regularly and even more. I exercise and try to watch what I eat. I am still taking prescribed vitamins, acidophilus and antioxidants. I try avoiding stressful situations or people. I try to keep up with current information.

(Heather Resnick, Thornhill, ON, diagnosed in 1997 at age 43, recurrence in 1999)

I regularly go for checkups, blood work, and chest X-rays. I read about new research on breast cancer or recent findings to be continually informed. I feel discouraged to hear someone has died from breast cancer as I'm sure most of us are, but I certainly do not want to know the details. I feel that if I wasn't true to BSE, I might have found it at a stage where it wasn't as treatable.

(Carolyn S. Olson, diagnosed at age 37)

I live life to the fullest for the moment, and I don't think too far ahead. I read positive messages and avoid talking about breast cancer. I don't want to be called a breast cancer survivor. I had breast cancer and now I don't.

(Yvette, Victoria, BC, diagnosed in 2002 at age 47)

I do not feel discouraged to hear of a death from breast cancer, but it does make me feel I must live each day to the fullest and take time for myself. Eat healthy and exercise daily and do not forget to pamper yourself weekly.

(Penny)

Having to go through it a second time (four years later) is very discouraging indeed. It was more difficult emotionally. I felt it was more serious because it was back, which made me feel defeated after all my efforts to change. But I had much better support from friends and now I was informed and "plugged in." I knew where to get help and support. I was 37, had just met someone I thought was the man of my dreams, and I was told I had to have a mastectomy. I had not told this man that I had previously had breast cancer, and I did not want the fun to end. He was very supportive but, after the mastectomy, he lost interest in me sexually. This is a very difficult rejection to get over.

(Donna Tremblay, diagnosed in 1992 at age 33, recurrence in 1996)

A total medical checkup once a year, a complete day in the hospital for all kinds of tests. That day, I think of recurrence. In everyday life, I don't think about it. I compare myself to the other women, and we all have the same chances of getting cancer or not. I'm optimistic. If ever cancer recurs, I will worry in due time, not beforehand.

(Annemie D'haveloose, Belgium)

My battle plan to cope with cancer has been to continue my normal life and consider myself healthy as long as nothing appears. It simply does not help at all to worry about what might happen. I now have cancer for the second time. I am happy that I lived happily for 4 years in between. My second treatments will be over this summer (2004) and I have already decided to continue my life as healthy again. The fact is that nobody knows what diseases are coming into your life, and they always come totally uninvited. Why worry beforehand?

(Katariina Rautalahti, Järvenpää, Finland, diagnosed in 1999 at age 41, recurrence in 2003 at age 45)

While I was going through treatment I was kept so busy I didn't have time to think. I felt in control because I was doing something about it.

The chemicals, the surgery, the radiation, but now all there is are these little white pills. How can they possibly be keeping the cancer away. I feel like I'm on a ledge ready to fall off. Only someone who's been there knows what I'm feeling.

(Linda Bryngelson, New Brighton, MN)

Recurrence happened 14 months later. A local recurrence does not in itself worsen the prognosis. No two tumors are exactly alike. Therefore everyone's story is different. Don't compare yourself to others. Just do everything you can to live a healthy lifestyle.

(Shelagh Coinner)

I get scared when I hear someone has passed away from breast cancer. Recently I dealt with first death within the support group. It's hard.

(Cordelia Styles, Quesnel, BC)

It's important for women to know the geography of their own breasts so that they can recognize changes and get help. Recurrence in same location in 2001, found on mammogram. I had a second lumpectomy on the same breast, contrary to the usual recommendation in this country. Hearing the news the second time was much easier.

(Bev Parker, Naperville, IL, diagnosed in 1985 at age 40, recurrence in 2001)

Every time I get an ache or pain anywhere in my body, it's back. This I understand will never go away. Mammograms sure helped me, and I wished I had had one sooner.

(Jacqui, Courtenay, BC, diagnosed in 2002 at 38)

What triggers the fear? I think anyone who has experienced a life-threatening disease of any kind secretly wonders about recurrence, not all the time but it's there, in the back of her mind. I know my body now, and if I think there's something that needs looking at, I will not stop until I get the answers.

(Rebecca Simnor)

I definitely believe in mammograms, and I always ask for the radiologist to be there to read it before I leave. That always eases my mind.

(S.R., Columbus, OH)

My regular checkups always trigger my fear of recurrence. I think most women feel blindsided by their diagnosis. They go to the doctor feeling perfectly fine and come out with a life-threatening disease. If it can happen once, it can happen again.

(Rita, Palos Verdes, CA)

I have a very strong fear of recurrence. Because doctors are unable to give you definitive guidelines or predictions, you always wonder with every little pain if it's recurred. It is difficult to treat Her2Neu+ breast cancer and the prognosis is fairly grim because it is so aggressive. Although when I write this it seems frightening and exhausting to have to endure such a treatment, I looked at it as relentless attacks on my cancer and was actually more frightened when it all ended.

(Catherine, Pointe Claire, QC, diagnosed in 2001 at age 39)

13 years later, I found a lump in my other breast. I enjoy helping others who are recently diagnosed. I like telling them my story and giving them courage. Always believe you can fight this. Half the battle is believing you can overcome this. I become fearful when I have a mammogram, I become fearful when I have a checkup.

(Marie, Co. Mayo, Ireland, diagnosed in 1987, recurrence 13 years later)

My fear of recurrence is not centered around the possibility of death, but around the possibility of having to go through treatment again. I don't know if I could consent to chemo again, so it's a fear of causing my own death because I'm too chicken to do anything about it. I hate it whenever I hear of anyone getting cancer or dying of cancer. I work in a hospital, so this is constantly in my peripheral vision.

(Judith Quinlan, diagnosed in 2001 at age 52)

Fear is an important element of the equation of breast cancer. I see fear as the factor that gets us in touch with our strength. Fear serves as the backdrop for what we are trying to learn or to overcome. I found that by realizing what my greatest fears were that I knew where I needed to start my healing journey. Death was my greatest fear of breast cancer. I had to learn about death, and what and why I was so afraid of it. Once I learned about death, fear had no hold over me. I found that I was actually starting the first and most important step of the healing journey by seeing I couldn't heal while I was bound by my fears to make decisions from a place of fear. I was regularly making decisions from a foundation of fear, instead of from a place of empowerment.

(Beverly Vote, Lebanon, MO, diagnosed in 2002 at age 37)

I used to fear finding a lump, but now I fear more missing a lump. Once you've been through this, you really understand the benefits of early detection.

(sams mom)

I have over 200 books on breast cancer and positive thinking. I like to read all I can about it. I do think about it coming back but do not dwell on it. I feel self-exams are important. If I hadn't done mine I would never have found the lump.

(Marianne Svihlik)

The outcomes are different for all of us. I remain optimistic and hopeful that the years of good lifestyle/eating/exercising, etc. will keep me healthy. I think women should be encouraged to do self-exams.

(Lorraine)

Whenever I hear that someone has died of breast cancer, I automatically want to know her estrogen receptor status, her type of treatment, and how long it's been since her initial diagnosis. Since I'm active in the Young Survival Coalition and on the WebMd boards, I've known several women who have died, which just makes me want to fight harder for a cure. I don't think mammograms are effective in women under 40. My tumor was over 2 centimeters, and it didn't even show up on the mammogram. Luckily it was painful, so I knew that something was there. An ultrasound located it.

(Leslie, Springfield, VA)

I will not let myself give into this fear. I prefer to focus my efforts on maximizing every day God gives me on earth. I have been given great gifts of intelligence, compassion and humor. I do not dwell on breast cancer nor do I take my identity from this disease. I regard it as a "speed bump" in life and have moved on. I spend my time working for volunteer causes in my community and singing. I found my voice again after 15 years of not using, and I'm going to sing as long as I can.

(Mary Schmidt)

My fear of recurrence comes from my sister. She is a six-year survivor of breast cancer but metastasized 11 months following her original diagnosis. That had put fear in me. I read lately that they want women to have a mammogram every two years, instead of every year. I will challenge anyone who says that a yearly mammogram doesn't help. Early detection helps.

(Dawn, North Hollywood, CA, diagnosed in 2001 at age 47)

Fear isn't useful except as a motivator of positive action. Be happy, have more fun, eat better, love more, be grateful for all the beauty in the world, forgive and forget...

(Anonymous)

I was raised on the Saturday morning cartoons of "Schoolhouse Rock" and always remember "knowledge is power!" We can't live in fear, we have to be proactive. Self-exam is what found mine, so I truly believe in that. I wish doctors were more aggressive with mammograms for women under 40, like myself.

(Lori Hughes, diagnosed at age 35)

My battle plan is to become as healthy as possible in all the things I can control. I can't control cancer, but I can control what I eat and whether or not I drink alcohol or smoke. I eat lots of fruits and vegetables. I no longer eat red meat, and I exercise regularly. Soreness in my breasts makes me nervous. I have to take a deep breath before I do breast self-exams or before I get a yearly mammogram.

(Julie, diagnosed at age 26)

After 30 years I still feel a little apprehensive when it's time for my yearly checkup with the breast surgeon..... I know it can happen again. However, I have lost the excess weight, go to the gym five days a week, and I am fit for the first time in my life. I stopped smoking in 1974 when diagnosed with cancer. I eat right and take antioxidants. I feel great and no longer fear that I will die of cancer. My mother died at the age of 41 from uterine cancer so when I got cancer at 41, I needed several months of therapy to get over that fear. I am a very happily married artist and keep a very busy schedule. I take care of myself these days.

(Gloria J. "Mimi" Winer, Point Pleasant, NY, diagnosed in 1974))

I am scared to death of recurrence. My mother-in-law recently died from advanced stages of breast cancer, and it was very hard to take. I try and deal with things in a positive manner, but sometimes you just have to cry!

(Peggy Scott, Waldorf, MD, diagnosed in 2002 at age 46)

Any ache or pain triggers unspoken fear of recurrence. I don't know any survivor who doesn't experience this. My battle plan is to eat well, laugh a lot, and make the best of each day.

(Joan Fox, Victoria, BC)

Women have to realize that not feeling a lump doesn't mean they don't have cancer. I had no lump.

(Cheryl Otting, Elkford, BC, diagnosed in 2002 at age 53)

In the first few years, I was very fearful. About four years after, a routine mammogram found what they believed were calcifications in my right breast... and, until the biopsy results came back, I was a real nut case! If I hear someone has died of breast cancer, I think how very fortunate I am to still be here.

(Christine)

I feel like I have a sisterhood with these women and I feel the loss when one of us is taken. I am not afraid to hear the stories.

(Deborah, diagnosed in 2002 at age 46)

My doctors have made it very clear that I am at a very high risk for recurrence so I deal with fear every day. It's hard.

(Jennifer, diagnosed in 2001 at age 27)

What triggers my fear is when I feel overtired and stressed. I became acutely aware of the passing of time and what is meant by quality of life. I weeded out friends who were exhausting and dependent. I became more aware of my nutrition. I spent less time cleaning my apartment and more time out in the country, hiking, cycling, walking, exercising. I cut back on my work hours. I am strapped a bit financially, but it is worth it. I get impatient with people who want to delve in details and who take up too much of my time for no good reason.

(Donna Tremblay, diagnosed in 1992 at age 33, recurrence in 1996))

I worry that it may come back. I want all tests done every six months. Oncologists do not want that, saying that they think it creates more stress. They do not realize that with every clear test, it leaves us with hope that we made it one more time. And if it is not a clear test, why not know as soon as possible and hopefully do something about it? The mammogram missed my cancers. We have to find a better way to diagnose.

(Sharron, diagnosed in 2002 at age 62)

My recurrence began with a pain in my side when I would roll over in bed, with a few back pains thrown in. It was exactly two years after I had completed the initial treatments, and I had been on tamoxifen. The bone scan revealed the metastasis to the ribs, vertebrae, and hips. There is a lack of knowledge about metastasis and the emotional ups and downs we go through. The biggest comment everyone gets from friends is, "But you look so good!" My online support group has constant discussions about this, as it is frustrating to everyone. Living with the constant fear and knowledge that your time on earth is limited and you need to make the most of it right now, is somewhat of a struggle. That is true for the whole population, but having the reminder "in your face" daily is a challenge. Making plans even six months ahead is difficult as you always wonder, "Will I still be feeling well by then?'

(Jane Sterett)

Staying busy and occupied was very helpful. I didn't experience depression until after all the treatments. Seemed like when the treatments were over all the constant attention came to an abrupt halt and everyone (in medical support) went away. I felt alone and scared. I don't know if I will ever not wonder if it is back every time I have a weird pain or symptom.

(psh)

I just hope that if it does happen, it's somewhere in the future when there will be a cure.

(Leslie, Springfield, VA)

Each day this disease kills many women who might have been saved by regular breast exams or mammograms. An annual mammogram is inexpensive, an appointment will take less than an hour of your time, and it could save your life.

(Barbara Brabec)

Fear of recurrence is so huge... it gets in the way of believing that you have a future to plan. Service to others helped a lot. Getting involved in public education about breast cancer, in Race for the Cure and working with other survivors helped me tremendously.

(Janel Dolan Jones, Fort Worth, TX)

My first breast cancer was eight years ago, the second was four years ago, and I recently have been diagnosed with another recurrence. My first warning sign was pain in the sternum for over a year, not necessarily typical. A PET scan showed a bright area over the sternum but nothing showed on MRI so it was decided this was just some sort of inflammation. The pain persisted but my oncologist felt it was just part of the healing from the reconstruction. Then my husband and I noticed a fullness or raised area, another PET scan showed a larger area of brightness, and a CT scan confirmed a mass invading the sternum, ribs and pectoralis muscle along with an internal mammary node. Because I work in the oncology field as a radiation therapist, I see a lot of situations. It can be scary to see young women come in with recurrences. But I also know of women who had recurrences 10 to 15 years ago and no one thought they'd be around, and they're still going strong. I plan to be one of those women.

(Joni)

Optimism and Pessimism

What helps you to cope

If it rains, let it rain, if wind blows, let it blow. (Ikkyu)

I read many years ago that after a profound crisis like the death of a loved one, a divorce, or a life-threatening illness, you will eventually recover the personality you used to have. That became another lifeline to give me hope since my basic personality is optimistic. A positive attitude got me through many tight turns in life. "I refuse to die," I declared in the midst of my cancer, and one of my doctors smiled and said that an attitude like that will help me more than I can imagine.

In retrospect, after surviving it, even a cancer journey can be an interesting experience. I believe that our cells obey our feelings. To boost my positive thinking during the treatments, every night before falling asleep, I read a few pages of The Power of Your Subconscious Mind, and counted my reasons for gratitude. I was rewarded with the most beautiful healing dreams.

I can affect my mental attitude and this simple truth works wonders: if I think negative, it gets worse, and if I think positive, it gets better. Accepting fear and anger as soon as it happens helps me to be positive. Expecting always to feel positive is stressful and unreasonable for anyone but especially for the cancer patient. The moments of sadness and distress found their way into my cancer journal and are now mostly forgotten.

Dwelling on the negative simply contributes to its power.
(Shirley MacLaine)

Accept support from friends, family, and coworkers who let you be you.

Share your feelings.

Allow yourself to feel fear, anger, anxiety, self-pity, and sadness to release the tension, and to make room for optimism.

Discover the power of a good cry, humor and laughter.

Reach out for spirituality, including prayer.

Start journaling to accept your feelings.

Get connected with a peer support group to keep motivated and active in pursuing the best treatment plan, and to get through the treatment process, both emotionally and physically.

I needed to move toward hope, spirituality and seeing what could come from the experience, because that is who I am, and it is how I move through life. But I also had many terrifying, sad and angry moments. People need to express the whole range of human emotions they have, and they need to be true to their way of dealing with life—not pretend and push away the dark feelings. Ultimately I think that hurts your body.

(Lorraine Langdon-Hull)

Cancer is a disease of toxins, which includes emotional toxicity. Fear is one of the biggest toxins in our life, and by removing or changing our perspective about fear of breast cancer, we remove what feeds the cancer's growth.

(Beverly Vote, Lebanon, MO, diagnosed in 2002 at age 37)

Stay positive by expressing your feelings as best you can. Don't try to be cheerful if you are not feeling so. Be whatever you feel you are. Walking with friends helped keep me positive and connected with my world. We'd talk about work and writing and things other than cancer, but I'd talk about cancer if I felt like it. It was much better than sitting inside and talking, and between chemo sessions I needed to have someone to walk with in case I fainted.

(Maria Hindmarch)

The ability to look at others and see there are so many that are worse off was helpful to me.

(Joy McCarthy-Sessing)

I am fortunate to have always been a positive person and this was no exception. If you are experiencing fear or anger that is in any way incapacitating, seek counseling. It is always good to talk to someone who can be an objective listener, especially someone familiar with the subject. A positive attitude makes the journey a lot easier.

(Shelagh Coinner)

I don't want to be treated as a celebrity for surviving, and my family and friends understand that. There are people that risk their lives, volunteer, do special things for others that we never even know about; they're the heroes, and I strive to be like them. Having breast cancer made me realize that I am loved beyond my imagination.

(Rebecca Simnor)

I think positivism is bullshit. I hated it when people said to me that I should keep a positive attitude or even complimented me on being so positive. Why should you feel positive? Anger and humor were my best defences and still are. Depressing? You betcha! Self-pity? Why not? Self-blame? Not on your life. Stress? After breast cancer everyday stress is nothing.

(Judith Quinlan, diagnosed in 2001 at age 52)

Take it one step at a time. Don't look at the big picture but the little steps along the way.

(Linda Bryngelson, New Brighton, MN)

I always worried that my stress or pessimism would bring on a recurrence. I was recently relieved to read a study that shows no connection to recurrence. I am angry and depressed but find that as time goes by, I don't always think about it 24/7 like I did the first year. I would like to celebrate each year with a big party but

Read books about coping, and about emotional and physical issues relating to a cancer diagnosis and treatment.

Listen to inspirational and motivational tapes.

Do something with passion.

Make a gratitude list of what's good in your life. Appreciate what you have.

Realize that there are worse things than breast cancer.

Discover what makes you feel better. Emotions may fluctuate from moment to moment; this is normal.

Use professional help with antidepressants and counseling for prolonged depression and sleeplessness.

Complementary treatments (page 107) might help you cope with pain and distress.

---

still feel too nervous to do so. So I quietly say a prayer of thanks on my anniversary. I try to be aware of every good moment I experience.

(Catherine, Pointe Claire, QC, diagnosed in 2001 at age 39)

Let yourself enjoy your life and put your fears aside as often as possible. Suddenly it becomes a pattern and it makes your life easier and happier.

(Katariina Rautalahti, Järvenpää, Finland, diagnosed in 1999 at age 41)

I do allow myself to feel low every once in a while but only for a day or two. I think after all we have been through it is okay.

(pmc)

You only have two choices: Be happy with breast cancer or unhappy with breast cancer. I choose to be happy. I have so many blessings in my life and things to be thankful for that I focus on them rather than being sad. I think that this kind of optimism can be learned. I just focus on the next happy moment and try to spend more time with family and friends. Despite all this, I do have my moments. If my husband is traveling and I'm alone with my thoughts, my mind can wonder to places that are very unpleasant.

(sams mom)

Helping others always helps me. I enjoy talking with others and sharing my story. People are inspired to hear I have battled this twice in my lifetime.

(Marie, Co. Mayo, Ireland, diagnosed in 1987, recurrence 13 years later)

People were telling me how brave I was. I never felt this way, I simply felt the option of curling up in the fetal position and crying was not going to help anything. Blaming yourself or God or whatever also does no good. I figured I would gain as much control as I could by at least being in charge of my emotions. Was I scared? Hell yes, but I also always remained optimistic. I have a toddler that needed her mommy. I didn't have the option of skipping out emotionally.

(Julie Austin, Little Rock, AR, diagnosed in 2000 at age 30)

Both optimism and pessimism have played a role in my surviving cancer. It is a long haul and I was not happy all the time. I was optimistic that what I was doing was the very best I could. Yet within that optimism comes the depression from all the physical changes that occurred to my body—the sleepless nights, the anger and irritability from being overwhelmed and taking the steroids, the fatigue, self-pity, the fear that the treatment may not work, the fear of death and pain, and the frustration of trying to lead a normal life while all the chaos of the treatment is around you. I still struggle with depression and anger, and I go to counseling to discover the root of these emotions and why they still linger.

(Dikla, North Hollywood, CA)

I am a very positive person. Life is too short to worry over something I cannot control. If cancer shows up, then I can take care of it, one way or another. But to sit and think each and every pain is the return of cancer, well, that is time ill spent. Of course, I fear it will return, but my days are for the living. When I wake up in the morning, I can do anything I want. . . I am a woman.

(Gwyn Ramsey)

I think what I like most about posting on the Internet is that I can express exactly what I'm thinking or feeling without fear of being judged. My family was not terribly supportive of my ups and downs. I wish they had reacted differently, but at least I had an outlet on the net. The ladies at Healingwell.com are truly friends.

(Rita, Santa Clarita, CA)

I spent a lot of time in my garden, which I found very therapeutic.

(Dawn, Victoria, BC)

Feel sorry for yourself as often as you need to, but then get on with your life. Exercise is great for pounding out stress, even if it is walking the dogs. Remember to laugh. I can't stress the positive effects of humor enough. Find someone you can talk to about things. Write in a journal and keep in mind the journal is for your eyes only. It really does help to get the thoughts out of your mind. It is a release.

(Peggy Scott, Waldorf, MD, diagnosed in 2002 at age 46)

My husband and family were very supportive, but sometimes in an effort to help me, they said things that upset me. My dog and cat were a great source of comfort. They just snuggled up next to me, and didn't say anything.

(Anonymous)

I am a happy, happy person with an incredible sense of humor. I immediately joined a cancer support group where, instead of crying each week, we visit, we learn about each other's lives and we laugh... a lot!

(Dawn, North Hollywood, CA, diagnosed in 2001 at age 47)

Try not to sit around too much. Go outside, even for a little walk.

(Carole, Victoria, BC, diagnosed at age 57)

All of us die but not all of us really live fully.

(Janel Dolan Jones, Forth Worth, TX)

When people asked me how I could be so positive I simply said, well I have two choices: I can have cancer and be depressed about it or I can have cancer and enjoy life. In either case I have cancer, so I might as well choose to make the best of it.

(Julie, diagnosed at age 26)

I thought of myself as saving nine of my friends from getting breast cancer (if one in ten gets breast cancer).

(Esther Matsubuchi, North Vancouver, BC)

What helped me to have a positive outlook is realizing that I had two choices: I could lay down and succumb to cancer, or I could stand up and fight it. I chose to fight it. I choose life. I choose to view the glass as half full now, because life is truly too short. I live without fear in life and always ask for what I want. I figure the worse thing that can happen is someone tells me "no." I am seeking experiences I never thought of seeking before. I love life and hope to accomplish a great deal and make a difference in this world.

(Stephanie)

I joined a survivor dragon boat team and I've never looked back. I have more friends who are there for me than I ever had in my life. Having cancer has given me more gifts than I can possibly count.

(Joan Fox, Victoria, BC)

Keeping as much normalcy as possible in my life at a time when my health was turning me upside down was very important to keeping me focused on moving forward.

(Christine)

I used to vent my fears while in the shower, crying and getting angry at what had happened to me. That seemed to keep me on a balance, so I could deal with the reality of it next day. I did not need antidepressants or counseling.

(Amy Murphy, diagnosed in 2002 at age 32)

I wish I had spoken with a counselor sooner. It did help me to speak with a non-family member with an objective point of view.

(Kristina, diagnosed in 1995 at age 39)

I have become a more positive person and take nothing for granted. Problems are relative and I use my cancer experience as a reminder of what constitutes a really bad day. I am more likely to say what I feel and ask for what I want now. Life is too short.

(Alicia)

With all that I do, you would think that I am guaranteed to never get cancer again or at least catch it before it does any deadly damage—the truth is there are no guarantees in life. I trust my own instincts and I make all the decisions.

(Heather Resnick, Thornhill, ON, diagnosed in 1997 at age 43)

I have nine siblings and their encouragement and prayers helped a lot. I had my pity parties (weepy and anxious) and then I would dry the tears and do something uplifting like sit in my backyard and enjoy nature, listening to self-help tapes and music I love.

(Penny)

Cancer is my shadow. It is with me always. I would love for someone to tell me how to deal with the emotional and physical fatigue, since I haven't found an answer yet. I am on an antidepressant, and I have a counselor. I generally have a very positive attitude, but it's impossible not to be angry. It will be a while yet before I am able to really put this behind me.

(Jennifer, diagnosed in 2001 at age 27)

I think of myself as a realist. I am optimistic, but I don't want to put my head in the sand and not see reality either. This diagnosis was a real enlightenment in seeing how people deal with accepting this news. Many people are afraid to hear about it. Some stopped calling and only started calling after the treatment was over. I felt that I had to always be happy and optimistic with others and deal with other, more negative emotions such as fear, alone. The second time, four years later, my friends were very supportive and brought me through it. And I have learned who I can discuss my true emotions with, without upsetting them.

(Donna Tremblay, diagnosed in 1992 at age 33, recurrence in 1996)

After the treatments, I had a depression or something like it. I did not want any more medicine so I started running even more. Within 5 months after ending all my treatments, I ran the Copenhagen Marathon. When I ran, I could keep up the good spirit. I believe that exercising is very important if you tend to get depressed. If I should die before old age, I would like to say and for my family to say, "She was great fun and happy when she was here."

(Karen Lisa Hilsted, Denmark)

I surround myself with positive thoughts and people. I borrowed funny books and movies. My life is happy and complete, and I sleep well. I was determined not to live my life counting the days and years from my diagnosis.

(Yvette, Victoria, BC, diagnosed in 2002 at age 47)

Being able to sleep is a requisite for healing. Part of being able to cope was just leaving it all behind. I went camping with some women, nearly froze to death, but was able to not think about cancer for a few days.

(Sharron, diagnosed in 2002 at age 62)

It helped me a lot to go out, to see people, to dress well and to look good. I felt less like a patient then. I forgot my problems for a moment. I was back in real life and really enjoyed it. Then I lived more intensively than before.

(Annemie D'haveloose, Belgium)

I don't know if a positive attitude will add any days, weeks, or even years to my life. But I do know that it makes life more enjoyable, not only for me but for those around me as well. It's now 28 months later, and I'm still enjoying life to the fullest! (The initial prognosis was less than 3-6 months to live.) I still work full-time in my Healthy Exchanges endeavors, I still garden with a passion, and I still love doing things with my family, especially having my grandchildren stay with us on weekends.

(JoAnna Lund, DeWitt, IA, diagnosed in 2002)

Initially, I wrestled with what I could have done to prevent this, and realized that it was too late to change anything. I had to move forward and deal with this disease and overcome it.

(Lorraine)

Fear will magnify every negative you experience.

(Anonymous)

Optimism plays a huge role during the emotional roller coaster during cancer. A patient needs to be able to express those hard, difficult, negative feelings, and often this is better to do with someone outside the family who is not as close to the situation. I found that people like to be able to help but often don't know how best to help, so let them know specifically what you need. Don't be afraid to ask for help, whether it's with daily activities, needing a ride somewhere, childcare, meals, laundry, yard work, or just needing to get out of the house for a change of scenery, or having someone to talk to.

(Joni)

Aftermath

Looking back when treatments are over and cancer moves behind you

One should count each day a separate life. (Seneca)

At first I felt like a woodchip in the rapids. I felt a surge of relief when the surgery was over and the treatments began. When the crisis was over, my hair grew back, my missing breast was camouflaged, and I looked normal to others. Yet I did not feel normal. I felt lost and the aftermath felt more frightening than the treatments. My imaginary safety net of treatments and attention disappeared, others around me returned to their normal lives, the doctors gave routine checkups spaced increasingly apart, and I felt lonely and vulnerable. Emotional fatigue was the worst. I had taken my health for granted and only understood its value after I lost it. Suddenly, I was shocked to notice articles about breast cancer almost daily. I was jumpy and worried about every little pain. Unlike medical emergencies like a stroke or car accident, you have options in treating the breast cancer. This is both a blessing and a curse. How was I supposed to choose in rush what's best when frightened out of my mind, knowing nothing about breast cancer, and feeling the sinister cancer was growing inside me out of control? At first there were only a few merciful minutes daily when I did not think of cancer, but in time the minutes stretched into hours and then into days. The first year was the worst. Then it got better, although I still revisit the fear at times. I understand and accept that things will always be different. Cancer became a divider of my life before and after.

I watched a program about Christopher Reeve who was working hours every day just trying to move his finger a little bit and hoping to walk again. He was forever positive until the end. Yet here I was sitting, feeling sorry for myself after cancer, even though I was fully able to walk any time I wish. So I went for a long walk, counted my blessings, and put a star on my calendar. And soon more stars were added.

*Do not wait for ideal circumstances, nor the best
opportunities; they will never come.
(Janet E. Stuart)*

*We all have big changes in our lives that are more
or less a second chance. (Harrison Ford)*

I will never forget the date of my surgery. I try
to do something special on that day. Remember that breast cancer is not the death sentence
it was once thought to be. If you get too stressed
out, take it a day at a time. If this is too much,
then half a day or even hour by hour. It does
get easier as the years go by.

(Marianne Svihlik)

It's common to feel a letdown after treatments
are over. Most people expect to feel elated so
this comes as a bit of a shock. Cancer is a very
complicated disease. Don't try to look for a
cause. There is no one way to do it right. Try
things and see what works for you.

(Shelagh Coinner)

I now feel that I can talk more freely about my
cancers. In the past I never said anything because I was concerned about being labeled as a
"sick person" or a person that was weak. I think
all the publicity and education of the masses
has helped all of us discuss cancer and our personal experiences more openly. During my three
bouts with cancer, I watched the dust bunnies
grow in my house. That really bothered me
when I was younger, but you know, when I was
being treated for breast cancer, it didn't bother

SURVIVOR TIPS

**ALLOWING YOURSELF TO
MOURN**

Acknowledge the loss
of your breast/health/life
as you knew it. Allow
yourself to feel sorrow.
Allow yourself to feel
hope again.

FACING STRESS

Seek moments of quiet
solitude daily. Make a list
of what stresses you,
then find solutions.

EMBRACING LIFE

Adjust to life after
treatments. Cancer is
behind you. Nourish
your body, mind, soul,
and spirit. Discover
things that give you
pleasure. Be self-
indulgent.

**TAKING A BREAK
FROM CANCER**

Work, hobby, book or
video will distract you so
you won't think of cancer
all the time.

JOURNALING

Journaling is
therapeutic.

EXERCISING

It relieves stress. Walk with a friend, with kids, with the dog, alone.

___

LAUGHTER AND TEARS

Allow yourself to feel authentic emotions.

___

MUSIC AND ART

Dance all alone in your living room. Lie down, close your eyes, and listen to classical music. Visit an art museum. Enjoy handmade art. Make something unique with your own hands.

___

TALKING

Talk about your experience with other survivors. Volunteer and visit other women with breast cancer if and when you are ready.

___

BSE

Know your body. Learn to perform self-exams.

___

ITCHY, DRY SKIN

Dry body brushing. Shower. Good moisturizing lotion. Comfortable cotton clothing.

me at all. My advice to other women when they are diagnosed is, "If you don't feel comfortable with anything your doctor says, or you think a doctor has not treated you promptly, go to another doctor. Do not give up—life is fragile and beautiful."

(Joy McCarthy-Sessing)

Thinking back, as a mom of teenagers at the time, it's hard, because life doesn't stop. Finding time in their busy lives to try to talk to each child and have them understand was very hard. I prayed, worked on relaxation, visualization, and learning something about nutrition. It was almost Christmas time. I didn't know what the year would bring, but I knew I would have Christmas, so that is what I concentrated on. As adults, my children have all told me that they really didn't understand. I still did what Moms do, maybe only laying on the couch a little more.

(Rhonda Shreck)

No one told me the fatigue continues and attacks when least expected. No one told me that I'd lose so much more than a breast; I lost all sensation, libido.

(Deb Haggerty, diagnosed at age 51)

After cancer I decided to continue my life as before. I also decided that I can take new challenges. This was the reason I joined the Aconcagua expedition. Seven European women with breast cancer history climbed Mount Aconcagua in February 2004. Everybody reached her own summit. Mine was at 5400 meters. For me this was a miracle since I did it between my 3rd and 4th chemo. I wanted to show that cancer does not have to destroy your dreams.

(Katariina Rautalahti, Järvenpää, Finland, diagnosed in 1999 at age 41, recurrence in 2003)

I kind of date my life now as before and after diagnosis. It gives me a perspective. Many people won't reveal that they have cancer, but I don't think that is smart. The support I received from my friends and family was incredible. I always thought I was independent and self-reliant, but I learned to accept help from others. This was not only really wonderful for me, but the others also appreciated the opportunity to be helpful.

(Anonymous)

I'm not worked up about doing work anymore. That is the worst thing. When I am off work, I just want to play. Realistically, I can't play all the time. Somebody has to vacuum. It is only through discipline that I do my chores.

(Deborah, diagnosed in 2002 at age 46)

My breast cancer is genetic. I feel this gene was triggered by stress. Being a single mother and going to University is stressful. I spent so many years in a stressful situation that it became normal to me. Only now that I am away from the situation do I see how busy and stressed I was. I worry about my daughter who is now 15. Will she have the gene? Will she develop breast cancer? Will she pass the gene to her children? How will this affect her future? I am on long term disability, constantly worried about money, still in treatment, and still struggle with my daily chores. My doctor appointments and treatments

RELAX CAUTIOUSLY

Finding a change in your breast does not mean you have cancer, but get it checked by your doctor.

REDUCE STRESS

Walking, deep breathing, fresh air, and nature are better than pills. Put yourself first. Don't try to please others. Forget about perfection. Slow down. Enjoy moments.

MUSCLE STIFFNESS, ACHES AND PAINS

Swim, do yoga, stretch, walk, pamper yourself with bath and massage. Use a heatbag (page 91).

WATER THERAPY

Water is the "oldest of ointments." Sit by a waterfront. Surround yourself with water in a shower, bath, or pool. Listen to the rain. Visit a waterfall. Enjoy the sounds of a fountain.

PROFESSIONAL HELP

If you are going through rough times and cannot sleep, get counseling and a mild antidepressant to help you cope.

---

are endless. I wish I would have taken more time for myself prior to my diagnosis, but that was not a reality in my life. If I had known my cancer was genetic sooner I could have been involved in the "high risk screening clinic." I never even heard of the clinic prior to my involvement in the genetic testing. I also feel people would have taken my concerns more seriously because they would be aware of my high risk. I hope these things will be in place for my daughter.

(Kathy Reeve, North Vancouver, BC, diagnosed in 2000 at age 32)

I celebrate each year that is my anniversary. I just like to celebrate any anniversary, I think! Inner strength is a key to staying healthy and to become involved in things other than yourself that keep you busy.

(Rebecca Simnor)

It has been almost 18 years since I was first diagnosed with cancer. Every day is a marvelous day, and my life is full and rich. Several members in my family have had cancer, including my son. I would have done nothing differently. I am just happy to be alive and look forward to the future. Our son is still living and so am I.

(Gwyn Ramsey)

What is really strange about all this is the fact that I was one of about 12 people so far in my neighborhood to get some form of cancer, and I'm not the last. The day I finished radiation my good friend and next door neighbor got the diagnosis that she has pancreatic cancer. I keep wondering that had I bought a house somewhere else, would this be happening to me. It's a scary thought that my house or my property or environment did this to me. And it's all happening to people who have lived here 20 years or more.

(Linda Bryngelson, New Brighton, MN)

I still get choked up when I remember telling my 7-year-old son that I was sick. He had picked up on the mood in the home and had seen his father and me talking and crying. I didn't know how much to tell him so I just said I was very sick. He asked me if I had cancer, which surprised me because I didn't think he knew what that was. Then he asked me if I was going to die. I told him I was taking treatment and it would be a long year with me not feeling well, but I was going to try to get well again. I never knew before if I could endure a calamity. I never knew my potential for mental strength. I have become so absolute, so defined. I have come into myself in time to enjoy it.

(Catherine, Pointe Claire, QC, diagnosed in 2001 at age 39)

Going through breast cancer now for the third time, I'm not sure how to talk to my 2-year-old daughter about it so that she understands. She is very bright, perceptive and verbal. I know children are resilient so I'm sure she will be fine. I pray that this will be my last bout with cancer. I don't want my daughter to look back on her childhood and have memories of her mom always being sick or weak or unable to participate in her activities. I want to be a fully active mom for her and give her my best.

(Joni)

The financial part is the hardest for me. Since I was off for eight months, I went through my savings. Being single, that means I have no financial security now. It's just one thing after another. I think it might have been easier to deal with this whole process if I hadn't had to worry every month about bills and how long treatment will take.

(Rita, Santa Clarita, CA)

I have felt very strongly about talking and keeping open with others regarding my cancer. I love to have all my friends join me in Run for the Cure races and shake hands with survivors I meet along the way. I talk openly to those who ask about what I have gone through. One positive from the illness was I got back my reading habits.

(Roberta R. Nordby, Redmond, WA, diagnosed in 1984 at age 29)

I don't wear my cancer as a badge, but I don't hide from it. I tell the truth if asked, but I don't want to be identified as "Mary Schmidt, cancer survivor." I do think that what we are doing to our environment has something to do with this disease. Now, I take care to eat foods that I know are grown or raised well. I'm lucky to live in a farming community, and I know the people who raise our beef, pork and vegetables.

(Mary Schmidt)

Today, anyone that knows me knows that I had breast cancer and what I did. I have been known to pull up my shirt and show the results of my reconstruction. I cannot tell you how many women—friends and strangers and even a few men—have been surprised to see that I am not scarred or disfigured. In fact, some say that they wish their real breasts looked like my new ones do. There is nothing that I could have done to prevent my breast cancer. The only thing I have changed since is becoming an advocate of mammograms and openly talking about my experience. I was in an auto accident 31 years prior to my diagnosis, in which my breasts smashed against the dashboard. My cancer was in exactly the same area. The calcification on the other breast was also in that impact area. I had nursed our son for nine months and was just weaning him when the accident occurred. I wish that there would be more research on the correlation between trauma and cancer.

(Helen B. Greenleaf)

I was relieved. I wanted to move on. My hair, eyebrows and eyelashes are back. I'm feeling close to normal other than occasional bitterness in my mouth due to certain foods. I had worked for a health care company before starting my own business and was well exposed to information about breast cancer. I may have been more diligent about having mammograms more regularly. I believe my diet and lifestyle have had a positive impact despite the diagnosis. I was able to return to my routine and work more quickly than the surgeon had expected. For other women, I would recommend they seek as much information as they can before making decisions about surgery and treatments. I learned a lot through my research and continue to do so.

(Lorraine)

Just prior to my diagnosis there was a great deal of stress in my life. My husband had been very seriously ill and unable to work so we had no income. We had to sell our home and move. Following my surgery and radiation treatments I decided that from then on I would take at least 15 minutes a day just for myself and do something that I wanted to do. One day I started painting, first on old wine bottles and then wood, and I loved it. I read magazines and bought brushes and paints and just kept painting. That 15 minutes a day has now grown into a web-based decorative painting business that keeps both my husband and I busy. He builds all the furniture we sell and I hand-paint it all. Painting, doing something that I love and found I am good at, has become my therapy.

(Sherry Gaffney, diagnosed in 1989 at age 47)

I feel great. I don't quite have the same strength as I used to, but I feel fine. I have no problems discussing my cancer to anyone who is interested. I have found from the beginning that it made it easier for me to talk about it. The love my family has for me made me feel so important, so loved, that I had to fight this thing.

(Carole, Victoria, BC, diagnosed at age 57)

I spread the word that I am a cancer survivor. I'm proud of it. I fought hard to be here, and I continue to fight to stay around for a long time. I enjoy life and don't let the little things stress me out. In the grand scheme of things it doesn't matter if someone cut me off in traffic as long as it didn't cause an accident. I'm going to celebrate my 5-year anniversary in a few months and I'm trying to get all my friends and family together to do the National Race for the Cure event with me. That way we can spend time together and give something back to the Breast Cancer community at the same time.

(Julie, diagnosed at age 26)

Excessive stress, the environment, the food we are eating with so many preservatives, loaded with antibiotics and additives, surely cannot be healthy for us... I've also used a lot of sugar substitutes and have had an occasional diet soda or two. I wish I would have eaten less artificial sweeteners, foods with preservatives and refined sugar, and more organic and fresh foods. I also have been on antibiotics a great deal, took a birth control pill for over 20 years and I never had children, and I've read all that may also have contributed to contracting cancer. I was my own advocate, and I was a critical thinker during the time I was establishing my medical team and receiving treatments. All that and obtaining second opinions was key toward the successful outcome of my experience. I also advise women to network and find someone who is strong, positive, and assertive to be your mentor, guide, and friend.

(Stephanie)

It took me approximately eight years to recover from my wife Glenna's death. Same for my then 9-year-old daughter. My strongest advice to survivors would be to get some kind of counseling or grief therapy. I did not do that and wish I had for both myself and my daughter.

(Dr. Barry J. Barclay, St. Albert, AB)

I feel great now, considering I am in my early 50s. I could stand to lose some weight, but healthwise all is great. I feel good, look good, and I am optimistic that I'll live to be an old lady! I don't dwell on why I got cancer. I believe it had a little to do with a lot of variables, the water in this area, probably my diet. I have always had weight management problems but I doubt if I would have done anything differently, and except for eating more "good" foods, I haven't really changed anything.

(Christine)

It's impossible for anyone to understand what one goes through with the mastectomy, chemo and radiation unless you've been there. I wouldn't have understood if someone tried to explain it to me. I don't celebrate the anniversary of diagnosis, but I do celebrate the anniversary of my operation to remove the cancer. As far as I'm concerned, the rest (chemo and radiation) was preventive maintenance.

(Joan Fox, Victoria, BC)

I never had pain due to the cancer. I just had pain due to the surgery and the healing process. I feel I got cancer because I was overweight. After my cancer, I lost 122 pounds by just watching my diet.

(Marilyn R. Prasow, Long Beach, CA, diagnosed in 2001 at age 60)

I feel great to have gone the route of treatment that I took. It sometimes seems like it was a lifetime ago that this happened. I always keep my head up. I am a survivor. I speak up for myself more, and I am not afraid to question anything or anyone. Having cancer gave me this power I didn't know how to use.

(Kristina, diagnosed in 1995 at age 39)

I was a little nervous as well as glad that the treatments were over. I was nervous because now that I am done, the doctors are not actively treating me anymore. I feel that my cancer was in part due to a lot of stress. I did wonder what I did wrong with diet and lifestyle, but the oncologist says some things we have no control over. So I continue to eat right, exercise and pamper myself more often now. Word of caution: reading too much about breast cancer can at times make you more anxious and worried about your situation.

(Carolyn S. Olson, diagnosed at age 37)

The most difficult part, the time when I felt most alone and not understood, was when the treatments were over and I was expected to be back to normal. Normal became something else and I had to find a way to find out what my new normal would be. During the treatment period, people were calling me and visiting often, then it came to an almost abrupt stop as everyone got back to their own life, saying "it is over"— but I was left with a strange feeling of insecurity.

(Donna Tremblay, diagnosed in 1992 at age 33, recurrence in 1996)

I am convinced that body and mind are one and whole. I think that's what cancer made me realize. I got cancer in a turbulent period of my life, a period in which I demanded too much from my body. I didn't sleep enough, I was physically exhausted, but I continued my life. Now I know that I have a body that I have to respect. I listen to it. I had to learn to enjoy sleeping. It was hard to do, because to me, sleeping was a waste of time. Now I pamper myself and tuck myself in. And I take care of the food I eat.

(Annemie D'haveloose, Belgium)

Very tired a year after chemo. Since then, I had a major surgery, two blood clots in leg, shingles twice, my son left home for college, I went bankrupt, and moved to a small apartment. Then I broke my shoulder. Now I eat very healthy and try to walk. Am I happy? You bet!

(Cordelia Styles, Quesnel, BC)

The first book I read after my second cancer was Christopher Reeve's *Still Me*. It was full of inspiration and hope. Then I read the story of Terry Fox. I attend breast cancer workshops all the time, and there is a clear link between diet, stress and the environment and breast cancer.

Learning how to effectively deal with stress, controlling our diets and proper exercise will make a difference.

(Heather Resnick, Thornhill, ON, diagnosed in 1997 at age 43)

I felt anger. Why me, why now when I just started my own business, when I am too busy and have so many interesting things ahead? I was comforted that my sister had gone through breast cancer and felt almost guilty that hers was more serious than mine. I prayed in distress and promised to devote myself to volunteer work if I survive. I have conveniently forgotten my promises and life goes on. What more can I ask?

(Maarit)

Calls from friends and family space out and they start making comments like "it is over." But it wasn't over for me. The treatment was the only thing that was over.

(Jennifer, diagnosed at age 27)

Knowing what's ahead will relieve a lot of stress, so ask straightforward questions. Develop a positive attitude. And focus on things other than your disease.

(Barbara Brabec)

I don't know why I got it, it's just something that happened. I don't believe there is anything in my lifestyle that contributed to it, I did not bring it on myself. The anniversaries have all passed without remarks, I have mostly forgotten the dates.

(Dawn, Victoria, BC

I feel great right now. I have never felt better. I still see the oncologist every six months for three more years so that makes me feel good that I am checked thoroughly. There are so many factors that contribute to cancer: chemicals, pesticides, food additives, stress, diet, alcohol. Breast cancer is a very slow-growing cancer. I believe it started when I was in a destructive marriage. Young women need to be educated about breast cancer and how to prevent it.

(Sheryl)

(Back in 1974...) The Cancer Society sent a little old lady to visit me. She brought me a bra and a soft lightweight prosthesis to wear at home. I could not relate to her. I wanted to talk to someone like me, never found her. I became afraid to meet men. I became hostile so they would not hang around, and I would not have to tell them about my surgery. This went on for a couple of years until I finally met a really nice man, and it became time to tell him about my surgery. His reaction was wonderful, "Oh hell, I thought you were going to tell me you had your period." That was a happy time, I discovered that if any man, and there had been several, had a problem, it was simply his problem, I was more than a breast. Too bad it took so long to figure it out. Before long my surgeon had me visiting other single young women in the hospital having mastectomies. I did this for several years. My then boyfriend, now my husband, usually went with me, and the women and their men had more questions for him than for me. They basically wanted to know if there was sex after mastectomy. Of course there is, eventually you get comfortable with who you are. Several months, even years after surgery you will feel pain, severe pain lasting for only a second, and it is frightening until someone tells you that these pains are announcing that those nerve ending have come back to life. This continues for a few years, and eventually when you feel one you just say, "Welcome back, you have been missed."

(Gloria J. "Mimi" Winer, Point Pleasant, NY, diagnosed in 1974)

I don't know how I got cancer, and that's one of the mysteries. You can guess all you want, no one knows. Scary. The only thing that I would do differently before my diagnosis of cancer was to have a mammogram before kids and after each kid. I think my cancer would have shown up and perhaps we could have avoided chemo, but this is wishful thinking on my part.

(Jacqui, Courtenay, BC, diagnosed in 2002 at age 38)

My focus was on healing. As soon as my body had healed from surgery, I started doing very gentle exercises and then I would add more challenging ones. It was almost like taking baby steps and learning how to walk all over again. Slowly but surely. Then I started walking every day, no matter how sick I felt. I knew the walk and the fresh air would help to clear my head. I noticed that I was looking forward to my walks because they kept me focused on getting better. One day, in the middle of winter, I went for my daily walk, and on that particular day I enjoyed so much hearing the crunch of my footsteps on the fresh, clean snow. I felt the cold, brisk, winter air on my cheeks. It was wonderful to be out there, feeling again. I knew I was on the road to recovery.

(Modestina)

I celebrate every anniversary with flowers—this year two flowers with one for good luck!

(Lorraine Zakaib, Kirkland, QC, diagnosed in 2002 at age 49)

I was angry that nothing was done to prevent breast cancer. I was angry that women have so few choices available to fight the cancer and not one is a cure. I felt that I had to become an advocate for other women, to find my voice and speak out, as my mother had never been able to do that. I couldn't believe that researchers had not made any progress in finding the causes of breast cancer when it is well known that the soil, air, food, and drugs are polluted with chemicals, pesticides, hormones, and other carcinogenic products.

(Sharon Tilton Urdahl)

For recovery I listened to a relaxation tape and some music for five years when I went to bed.

(Esther Matsubuchi, North Vancouver, BC)

It seems backwards to me to depress and destroy your immune system at a time when you need it the most. I was so miserable with chemo that I opted not to have the fourth round. I took tamoxifen very reluctantly and decided 4 months into it that it was not for me. I took Raloxifen instead for another 3 months and then quit. Now I do yoga, I journal and eat better, and sometimes I exercise. I have trained to be a life coach and strategist and work with cancer survivors (in workshops, retreats and group coaching) to create a better life than before they were diagnosed. I just celebrated my 5-year anniversary.

(Janel Dolan Jones, Fort Worth, Texas)

Support

**What helps emotionally, physically, practically,
and best gifts, best and worst things to say**

Hold a true friend with both hands. (Nigerian proverb)

I needed to feel that I matter and would be missed. Safety nets emerged, and my children became my strongest support. My daughter, barely an adult at age 20, interrupted her studies to be my mom and caretaker. I cried easily those first weeks and would immediately burst into tears to see my son, 25, who no longer lived with me. He would just hold me tightly and then we talked. One of my three sisters in Finland quit her job and came to see me. I had separated from my husband a few years earlier but he too became a great supporter, and this was important to us all. A cancer crisis demands a lot from the whole family and affects everyone. I surrendered and let my family take care of me. They went through it with me, and they validated my need to feel fear and talk about it. Good friends were in my corner.

One kind word can warm three winter months. (Japanese proverb)

The support group was a great help, but I wish I had been referred to them at the time of my diagnosis, because I endured two months without any help.
(Lorraine Zakaib, Kirkland, QC, diagnosed in 2002 at age 49)

Don't be afraid to ask for help with meals, driving you or your kids to activities, or even just to keep you company. I was told so many times that my friends were so thankful to be included in my journey, and they felt like they had learned so much from me. They also told me how glad

> ## WHO CAN HELP
>
> ### FAMILY
> Great listeners and strong providers of practical help get united in times of crisis. Tell them clearly what you need. Helping you both emotionally and physically is their way of coping.

SUPPORT FOR FAMILIES

Sometimes, partners and other family members cannot cope and might need help themselves; there are support groups for them too. If this happens, reach out to others outside your family. Illness and pain can make a patient irritable and uncharacteristically impatient; some family members are better at dealing with this than others.

FRIENDS

You might lose some friends who cannot cope. Other friends and acquaintances who can, become even closer. And you make new friends, some lasting way beyond your journey with cancer.

SUPPORT GROUPS

Only someone who has experienced breast cancer can fully understand your emotions, fears, and everything you are going through. You'll find support groups at the hospital, community cancer centers, and in Internet chatrooms.

they were when I gave them specific things to do, because they wanted to feel like they were contributing something to me and my family.

(Peggy Scott, Waldorf, MD, diagnosed at age 46)

I moved back to Vancouver and joined Abreast in a Boat (a dragon boating group) and they showed me the light at the end of the tunnel. We were all in the same boat, so to speak! I have now retired to another city and have started a dragon boat team for breast cancer survivors here.

(Pat Eveleigh, diagnosed in 1995 at age 52)

For the first anniversary of our diagnosis, my roommate at the hospital and I gave our surgeon (the best surgeon in the world!) a cigar and we gave daffodils to the oncology room. This year, we gave our surgeon two chocolate boobs. Some friends had a hard time dealing with my diagnosis and didn't call much. I knew they were there and knew they would find their way back in their own time, and they have. I hated receiving flowers, as my house smelled like a funeral home. Spiritual books were warmly welcome. It seemed that I was so tuned into God, it was an incredible experience. So many wonderful things happened to me during this terrible time.

(Jacqui, Courtenay, BC, diagnosed in 2002 at age 38)

After treatments, I stopped at a friend's farm and found two puppies there. We already had two dogs but one of those puppies just tugged at my heartstrings. A couple of days later, my husband and boys and myself went back and brought one of those puppies home, on the pretense of it being the boys' dog. Well, Fred is my dog and he's helped me calm down when I'm uptight. He's such a loving animal. He even puts me to bed at night. He's a gift alright, and there couldn't have been a better one.

(Cheryl Otting, Elkford, BC, diagnosed in 2002 at age 53)

One of the most interesting events occurred when a couple that we socialized with frequently found out that my wife, Glenna, had cancer. We never saw them again. They were absent at her funeral. Neither of her parents visited her in hospital more than a couple of times even when it was clear she was dying and was in a palliative care ward.

(Dr. Barry J. Barclay, St. Albert, AB)

My husband bought me a swing for when I came home. That was the best gift. Almost all of my friends dumped me when I was diagnosed but then, they weren't real friends. I have made many wonderful friends through the breast cancer group and other Internet groups I belong to.

(Marianne Svihlik)

Tell your friends all about it and let them know exactly what you need. Find those friends who really do want to help, not just offer. Let them know if you want them to accompany you to chemo or to the doctor and take notes for you. I loved the friends who would just show up with meals, books, or stop by to visit. I was looking out the window one day and saw two of my friends planting flowers in my yard! I was very open about everything and, because of that, felt that I had lots of people reach out to me. The more women know about what you are going through, the more they will respond to you and

---

DRAGON BOAT GROUPS

They are all breast cancer survivors, supporting each other, focusing on getting well and enjoying life.

COWORKERS AND EMPLOYERS

You are fortunate if your coworkers and employer are supportive and understanding, and if you feel comfortable revealing your illness to them.

CHURCH

Whole congregations are known to pray for their members.

DOCTORS, NURSES, TECHNICIANS

The best of them give you not only great medical care but also compassion and personal caring to make you feel safe and valued.

ANYBODY, ANYBODY

You need someone you can trust, willing to talk and listen. They respect your need to talk about cancer. They understand that sometimes you don't want to talk about the cancer, and sometimes you don't want to talk at all. Good listeners don't push their opinions and solutions when you are trying to listen to your own mind in the cancer jungle.

PETS

With unconditional love and acceptance, they make you feel needed.

INTERNET DISCUSSION GROUPS

They are supportive and anonymous, and you can be totally honest in the privacy of your home. Protect your privacy and use a screen name. Do not change your treatments or use alternative treatments based on their tips.

NEIGHBORS

You might discover a new friend next door for mutual benefit.

help you out. I have seen women try to "hide" their cancer diagnosis and never get the support they need.

(Jane Sterett)

Best gifts received? Unconditional love and encouragement from friends and family. My former boss said this to me as well, "The resolve of the type of person you are is not made by that which is handed easily to you in life, rather, it is that which you must face with some difficulty and fight for." Second best gift was a plaque from my sister with an engraved plate stating it was my one-year anniversary as a survivor.

(Stephanie)

The best gift I received was a big basket filled with my favorites, put together by a friend who collected over $300 from coworkers in the building where I work. It was filled with wine, cookies, candy, nail polish, body lotions, cologne, magazines, gift certificates for restaurants... it was just wonderful!

(Christine)

Along came cancer with great friends from a wide-ranging area. My husband ran while I walked in the first Run for the Cure. It was physically and emotionally the longest walk that I have ever taken. I volunteered for that organization the following year. I am now in my fifth year of paddling with the Two Abreast Dragon Boat team. We are a group of women and one man celebrating life after breast cancer and taking our message to the world through paddling. Last year seven of us from this team joined other

Canadians to create the Canadians Abreast Team and paddled in Auckland and Wellington, New Zealand. In April four of us will again join the national team to compete in the International Regatta in Cape Town.

(Vivia Chow)

Recovering from breast cancer was not an easy journey. I am so grateful to my family and friends for being there when I needed them most. Thoughtful gestures made the days that much easier to get through while I was going through my treatments. One of my best friends would make sure I received a big envelope full of encouraging mail from my coworkers. She sent me a package every time I went for a chemo treatment, and I would look forward to reading and rereading those uplifting cards. I do believe they got me through some of my darkest days. Now that's healing medicine for me!

(Modestina)

One neat thing that my friends did for me was a "Happy Everything Party" a few months after my radiation. I went through the major treatments from mid-October through mid-March so we celebrated all the holidays that I missed at that party. Trick-or-treaters came to the door, Santa came to see me, we had a toast on New Year's with noisemakers too, and my husband gave me a valentine. It was a lot of fun... and of course it was also a celebration that I had finished the toughest part of my treatment.

(Julie, diagnosed at age 26)

I don't go to support groups. I can't deal with seeing someone in an advanced stage of the can-

WHAT CAN HELP

PRACTICAL HELP FROM OTHERS

Going with you to the appointments. Making the appointments for you. With your consent, doing research on reputable web sites for the latest info and printing relevant articles. Running errands if you cannot drive while under medication. Taking care of your young kids, making meals, cleaning the house, shopping for groceries, checking up on you if you are alone.

FEEL-GOOD HELP

Compassion from others. Prolonged and profound hugs without words. Phone calls and emails from family and friends (saved correspondence becomes your journal). Talking about your ordeal and sharing it. Doing the breast cancer walk or run. Prayers by others. Visits from people whose company you enjoy. Cooking meals together and sharing them with friends. Freedom to vent your anger safely.

SELF-HELP

Focus on things that give you pleasure. Do something exciting. Read inspirational books about coping. Read interesting non-cancer-related books just for fun. Listen to Bernie Siegel tapes (mind-body lessons about self-healing). Watch good movies for entertainment. Put yourself first. Pamper yourself. Hot showers. Bubble baths with candles. Forgive others and yourself for past hurts. Be egoistic about your needs. Journal. Give yourself permission to be lazy and to do nothing at all.

PROFESSIONAL HELP

If the going gets too difficult, counseling and mild antidepressants might be needed to help you over the worst days.

RIGHT TO PRIVACY

Some prefer to keep quiet about their breast cancer and reveal it only to close family and best friends.

---

cer I have had. It is just too frightening for me. Let a puppy lick your bald head. I have a friend that I e-mailed almost every day during treatments; these are a journal of my experience.

(Alicia)

I have the best husband in the world. He looked after me and protected me to no end. He was at every treatment and every doctor's appointment. He looked after everything so I didn't have to. He was incredible.

(Jennifer, diagnosed in 2001 at age 27)

The very best gift that I got was the day that I was discharged from the hospital. My 11-year-old nephew had a baseball game that night and really wanted me to attend. I brought a chair to the game along with a pillow to rest my arm on. I was sitting directly behind the home plate fence. When Brandon came to bat for the 3rd time he walked in front of me, looked directly at me and said, "This one's for you, Auntie Cindy." With the count at no balls and 2 strikes he hit the ball so far out into left field that by the time the outfielder got to the baseball, my nephew was already on his way from third to home! It was a moment that I will never forget. I truly hope that someday he will understand what that particular moment meant to me.

(Cindy, Cedarburg, WI, diagnosed at age 41)

You cannot underestimate the importance of support. For me it has been the most important thing. When I have been falling down, my close ones and friends have spread a net where I have landed. I also think that support groups with the same disease history can help a lot.

These people really understand what you have experienced and can share your feelings. Humor is important but I have found that it is easiest to laugh with the members of my support group. It helps!

(Katariina Rautalahti, Järvenpää, Finland, diagnosed in 1999 at age 41)

My partner was in denial, angry, and took it out on me. We still haven't bridged the gulf this created in our relationship. This was the saddest thing about it all. Support came from elsewhere. I learned to lean on friends and avoid mentioning the C-word at home. Well, life ain't always fair.

(Judith Quinlan, diagnosed in 2001 at age 52)

I avoided the support groups, expecting them to be a venue where people gathered to cry about their disease and not be forward-moving. I couldn't have been more wrong. These people were instrumental in my support and sanity during the time of my recurrence. I found it therapeutic to sign up with two studies on breast cancer survivors and how they coped. These people wanted to hear about my experience. The more breast cancer meetings, lectures, and events I attended, the more plugged-in and empowered I felt. I became interested in a group described as a self-help group, for newly diagnosed breast-cancer patients. It was a series of five sessions, each with a different topic. I liked the formula. The bonds I made with the other participants are still there. The dynamics of the group were so good that we continue to meet twice a year in our 11th year.

(Donna Tremblay, diagnosed in 1992 at age 33, recurrence in 1996)

BEST GIFTS

USUAL BUT GOOD
Flowers and plants. Loving cards and thoughtful letters.

PAMPERING
Microwavable heatbag for comfort and pain relief (see page 91). Luxurious bath products and body creams. A recliner chair for lifetime of comfort. A dry body brush (one with a handle for back scrubbing). Gift certificates for a massage, foot care, or an osteopath. Exquisite chocolate. Heavenly cookies. Captivating novels to enjoy. CDs of good music for relaxing or dancing.

EMOTIONAL
Phone calls and visits. Truly listening to you anytime without giving unwanted advice. Prayers. A symbolic box of Kleenex. A small pocket stone etched with a word Healing. Guardian angels (small ornaments and pictures to surround you).

COMFORT CLOTHING

Comfortable button-up PJs to wear after surgery when everything else would hurt. A warm fleece blanket to crawl under. Large exquisite scarves. An extravagant hat or a goofy baseball cap for bald days. Soft cotton nighties (buttons on front or ties over shoulder when you can't lift your arms overhead, sleeveless for hot flash relief). Lovely loungewear for lazy days.

TOGETHERNESS

A drive in the country with a friend. Picnic lunch. Leisurely dinners with friends.

FOOD

Prepared meals. Gift certificates for restaurants. Invitations for homecooked meals.

UNFOLDING PLEASURES

A blank journal for private thoughts. A special trip when all the treatments are over.

All the details for treatments must have festered and when my husband arrived home, I had a full-blown tantrum, the very first since the initial diagnosis. I was so angry finally. And boy did I let it out. My husband tried to rationalize things with me but that didn't work, then he stood in a corner of the kitchen, well out of the way, and cheered me on. When I finished, I was spent and not at first but eventually started to feel better about what has to be. The next day when my husband arrived from work, he walked in the door and announced, "Your personal therapist has arrived." I was not able to join a survival group therapy due to distance so I was offered a telecommuting opportunity to be involved.

(Toni)

Lost no friends, gained many. The support person I called my first week of diagnosis was the one who helped a lot. I was able to help her as well when she had chemo, and we chatted many times on the phone before we finally met in person. That was the most rewarding, knowing I was leaning on her those first few weeks and that, even though I was still journeying through, I had energy and support for her in her time of need.

(Penny)

Having someone with you for appointments is mandatory. It took me a while, but I eventually came to realize it's okay to share your emotions, your thoughts and fears. It's okay not to have to be strong all the time, it's okay to let yourself be pampered, but most of all it's okay just to let yourself be loved. The network of support out there is phenomenal. My support group has been good for me, sharing my experiences with others travelling on the same train. Each step—the diagnosis, surgery, treatments—is like another car off the track. And so far, my train hasn't derailed! It's unfortunate that there aren't support groups in my area for spouses. They experience much of the trauma and go through a grieving process the same as breast cancer patients, maybe more in some cases.

(Virginia, diagnosed in 2001 at age 57)

I took part in the expedition "Beyond The White Guard" (women with breast cancer past climbed Mount Aconcagua in Chili-Argentina in 2004, http://www.BeyondTheWhiteGuard.org), the only time since my illness that I was surrounded by other women with breast cancer history. And it was a great experience. Some of these women have become real friends.

(Annemie D'haveloose, Belgium)

My friends made me a healing quilt with 120 hearts sewn together. They had sewing circles and met after classes in the school where our children were together. The quilt and a memory book were both presented to me the day before my first chemo began. I used that blanket each and every day after that. Each time I look at that quilt on my bed, I think of how loved I am.

(Dawn, North Hollywood, CA, diagnosed in 2001 at age 47)

I napped every day for half an hour or so. Before I napped, I put a red basket out on my front porch. After I napped, I brought it inside. Neighbors and friends knew that the red basket meant I was resting. A friend told me, "Don't read about cancer after three in the afternoon." This was

BEST THINGS TO SAY

"You are entitled," said my daughter when I said I am sorry for constantly complaining about feeling bad and scared. I was instantly comforted, my need was validated, and I felt great. "I won't let you die," she said when I started crying, afraid that I would never see flowers of another summer or my grand-children yet to be born.

"Tell me about it." It's therapeutic when people want to hear your story, truly listening to every detail.

My husband said my bald head was pretty.

"Don't worry, we'll take care of you," said my doctor when I needed many frightening tests.

"No, you won't die today, go out and play!"—said a doctor cheerfully about an innocent problem that worried me.

---

an excellent advice. Another friend told me on a walk, "Call me in the middle of the night if you want to talk." I didn't do it, but I knew she meant it and I could call if I wanted. Yes, I did stay away from some friends during cancer, those who demanded too much attention. My focus was quite inward. I didn't have the energy to help those who are more chaotic and dramatic. I do not live with my partner but he was supportive. When two doctors suggested that I could reduce the size of my remaining breast, he said, "Why monkey with a perfectly good breast?'

(Maria Hindmarch)

Emotionally, my support came from my friend across the street. She sent over food, sat with me when I was ill with chemo, listened to my rantings and held me when I cried, which was often. The relationships with many family members are very strained. Good thing we can pick our friends! The best gift I bought for myself was a good wig. I could not imagine myself going eight months with hats and scarves.

(Sharron, diagnosed in 2002 at age 62)

I started a support group that still meets today and those in it are among my closest friends. Volunteering in breast cancer groups gave me a reason for having had cancer; I couldn't repay all those who helped me, but I could pass that help and support along to others.

(Bev Parker, Naperville, IL, diagnosed in 1985 at age 40, recurrence in 2001)

I found my own support group of several women colleagues who had mastectomies, and whom I called "My Bosom Buddies." I lost closeness with one friend who had a lump at the same time. I urged her to have a biopsy because I was worried for her, but she felt I was thoughtless. Breast cancer was my worst fear, and now that it is realized, I have no fear.

(Yvette, Victoria, BC, diagnosed in 2002 at age 47)

The most helpful thing for me besides support from family and friends was to continue to fill my days with activities and people that have meaning for me. Eliminate what you don't like.

(Shelagh Coinner)

It was important to learn all I could from reading and from talking with others. My friends reacted differently. One couldn't come to see me; my illness scared her so much as I had always been so alive and strong. I had to reeducate my friends. I did find that there was a time when I had to move away from the support groups and the discussion groups, and from reading so much about the illness. I felt myself being kept in the illness by being immersed in it. There is a time to heal by moving away a bit.

(S.R., Columbus, OH)

I found out some of my friends couldn't deal with it and stayed away. I had one friend who made a dinner for four every time I had chemo since I wasn't hungry so my family didn't have to cook. I gained friends who have gone through the system and I value them.

(Marylynn)

I chose not to do chemo. I got two opinions from oncologists. One recommended chemo,

My husband called me endearingly a "pretty little noggin" after I lost my hair.

"You are the most positive person I know and I am sure it helps you through this difficult journey," said many.

...when anyone told me they loved me or laughed with me about the absurdity of it all.

...when a coworker told me how brave and strong she thought I was and that I was an inspiration to her.

"Don't read about cancer after three in the afternoon," said a friend. Another friend told me on a walk, "Call me in the middle of the night if you want to talk," and I knew she meant it.

...when a friend admitted she doesn't know what to say but that she is always there for me through everything.

"I want you to know that you'll never be home free. If the cancer metastasizes to other parts of the body, there is nothing more we can do for you," said one oncologist after my chemo. I thanked him politely but felt terror invading me. Then my wise daughter said, "How stupid! He should have said not to worry, and that even if the cancer does come back, there are so many things they can do, and more treatments are being discovered every day!"

They just had to tell me about someone they knew who was young, like me, with breast cancer, like me, and was dying. Did I really need to hear that?

"Breast cancer is nothing, I know many who have survived," said a friend when I told her my case is very serious.

the other didn't. I agreed with the reasoning of the second. However, I felt very defensive around many survivors who strongly feel one does "everything possible" without regard for the risks/gains ratio. I found an Internet forum established for breast cancer survivors. These people are supportive of whatever decision one makes. They are also there when I need to vent. They have been an important part of my recovery.

(Rita, Palos Verdes, CA)

My husband made sure that I went for a walk each day even when I really didn't feel like it, and I always felt better after the walk. And he put up with Oprah every afternoon. The ladies from my church were a wonderful support to me, they had a big party for me just after my diagnosis to let me know that they would be there for me. They also prepared a month's worth of dinners and filled my freezer, so when my husband wanted a night off from cooking he could pull a casserole from the freezer and dinner would be ready in about an hour with very little fuss. They also included several frozen desserts to satisfy my sweet tooth.

(Debbie Giroux, Langley, BC)

I had a heart-to-heart conversation with a wonderful woman who had experiences much of what I was feeling... some 12 years before. It was tremendously helpful, calming, and ultimately inspiring.

(Janel Dolan Jones, Fort Worth, Texas)

My last day before my surgery my coworkers took me to lunch and told me that they were doing "Walks for Women" the day before surgery and had raised nearly $1,000. That was so encouraging to me and told me that I was loved and that they were supporting me.

(psh)

My best support were my husband and three children, and also my daughter's boyfriend's mother who was diagnosed at the same time as me. I barely knew her but we had this bond that we shared, and we were there to help each other and shared tips. She sent over meals for the family on the days I had chemo. Every day even with my bald head my husband told me I was beautiful. One day after my hair had started to grow back I went shopping. At this point I was feeling pretty good, treatments were over, life was going on, and I felt great. But then I heard a little girl and her sister call me "the monster," I felt horrible, left the store and had a good cry.

(Linda Bryngelson, New Brighton, MN)

Faith, friends, keeping others' spirits up. One of my friends who had breast cancer flew down to be with me for my first chemo, and I was so touched.

(Deb Haggerty, diagnosed at age 51)

The support groups that I found seemed to be about expanding on how serious their cancer was and that it was more dramatic or more life threatening than everyone else's. I did not see a model for healing within the groups so I quit going. That is sad because we are not designed to heal alone.

(Beverly Vote, Lebanon, MO, diagnosed in 2002 at age 37)

"But I always told you that you are too fat," said a friend when I told her I have cancer. I did not need to hear it at that moment.

"Death is nothing to be afraid of, they'll give you morphine, and the afterlife is so much better than this crap here," said a friend. But I didn't want to die, not yet, and although serious, my prognosis was good.

"Oh, I suppose you'll change your lifestyle now," said an anesthetist as I was wheeled in to have a mastectomy.

"That means you are not ready to let go of your cancer," said a friend when I said that I am doing fine after one year, but sometimes still feel fear of recurrence.

I hated it when a friend acted as if I am dying right away, and another one dismissed my cancer as trivial.

After surgery, before chemo, a friend said, "It's over now!" That didn't make sense to me. This was the beginning. I still had that awful chemo to go through.

"Don't thank me for telling you you have cancer," said my doctor and laughed nervously when I thanked her. When I wanted to have the biopsy closer to home, she said, "Well, if you want us to just lop off your breast, we can do that here!" This was before my diagnosis.

"Such big, beautiful breasts, what a waste," said some women prior to my mastectomies.

I did not like it when people assumed how I feel or what they would do in my shoes. I wanted to tell them how I feel and what are my options.

"Oh my, well, that's something," said a friend of 20 years when I called her to tell I had cancer, and I never heard from her again.

With a small baby at home and a full-time job, I never had time to do a support group. But I found a tremendous amount of support from two bulletin boards (see end of book). After things settled a bit, I also was able to attend some events from the local chapter of the Young Survival Coalition. The most important thing was being in a room surrounded by happy, beautiful, vibrant young women who all seemed to be moving on with their lives.

(sams mom)

My support group provided emotional support as well as extremely practical information. My family helped me with research on the Internet and with my daily routine. They kept me motivated and provided a sense of humor. For some reason, surgery scared me more than chemotherapy. I was very, very nervous and anxious, and more so especially in pre-op. My group facilitator brought me a gift of a little stuffed blue bear with the statement "Cancer Sucks!" sewn into it. I loved it and it helped calm me down. It said exactly what I felt and was cute and cuddly to soothe me as well.

(Dikla, North Hollywood, CA

When I am asked to describe the whole experience in one line I can only say, "It was the best of times; it was the worst of times." (Charles Dickens)

(Susan, Brossard, QC))

My husband let me cry on his shoulder so many times. My teenage son told me straight out that he always wanted to know everything, and he didn't want me hiding anything from him. This really helped as I could go to him if I wanted to give my husband "a rest." The friend I took with me the day I went to try on imitation-hair wigs cried softly when I broke down in uncontrollable tears in the shop. I felt a lot of love because I saw that she was suffering just by seeing me suffer. I would have liked to see that with my husband, but he was determined to act strong in front of me. He would not want to hear of death or plans of what I'd like done in the future if I died. I told him that not wanting to discuss the subject was not helping me so he finally listened. I decided to look for an association for women with breast cancer and read up all I could on the subject. The association helped so much. I met women who were like me, which really helped a lot. I knew that there were others in the same shoes but I needed to actually see them. The exercises for breathing were great to learn, as they really helped me relax. I found a website (WebMd.com) and that gave me contact with others in my shoes without having to face them so I felt I could ask questions and let out my self-pity, etc. without being embarrassed. They had great tips to give me.

(Laura, Navarra, Spain, diagnosed in 1998 at age 41)

One of the things that helped me most was helping others. When you get out of yourself and share with another person and help them to go on, it makes a huge difference in your own recovery. During my second breast cancer, a friend was going through a much more serious type of cancer. The doctors gave her less than three months to live. She gave up emotionally. I sat with her and convinced her that there was a

I couldn't stand it when some friends started talking about their trivial aches and pains or the fights of their children when I told them I had cancer. This was my time. Finally I said I really didn't have patience to listen to their problems this very minute.

One thing I could never deal with was when people would come up to me and say, "I heard you were so sick." My answer was always an angry, "I'm not sick, I had cancer, but it's gone."

I was questioned why I didn't feel overwhelming fear and that I just don't recognize it and would have to deal with it later.

"But you look so good," said a friend and implied she did not believe I had a life-threatening illness.

A close friend, whom I love, said that 2.5 cm wasn't very large for a cancer.

chance. Eventually, she began to fight. Three years later she is still alive and in complete remission. Where there is life, there is hope. Stay strong and keep believing you can overcome this. Whatever you do, don't let it get you where you really live, in your mind. I received wonderful gifts of flowers. My daughter in the U.S. sent a photo of herself and her husband smiling that I brought with me for radiation. She also sent Frank Sinatra tapes that I could listen to. I danced while in the hospital and I laughed.

(Marie, Co. Mayo, Ireland, diagnosed in 1987, recurrence 13 years later)

I feel very lucky that I was not abandoned by anyone in my crisis. In fact, people came out of the woodwork to offer their support. Knowing people were praying for me and cooking for me and checking up on me made all the difference. During treatments there were periods when I didn't feel like talking to anyone for a couple of weeks. None of my friends took it personally and stuck by me through it all.

(Julie Austin, Little Rock, AR, diagnosed in 2000 at age 30)

I was a caring and compassionate person, sympathetic in the way I talked with cancer patients and their loved ones. Today, I have a different perspective of nursing, life, death, and cancer. I use the lessons I have learned from my own experience. I have experienced many of the same tests, decisions, side effects, and anxieties as the patients I work with. When I talk about the disease, I begin with the basics, even if I'm dealing with a healthcare professional. I don't assume anything. Once I became the patient, I was suddenly "dumb" and needed to hear everything in

> When people would say, "Keep positive," it would make me angry. I felt it wasn't up to anyone to tell me to stay positive. I felt I was doing my best.

> "Get your priorities straight," said an oncologist when I expressed sadness that I might never have children due to the cancer treatments.

> "Oh you poor woman," exclaimed a friend in horror when I told her I had breast cancer, and then she started telling me how many women die every year from this disease. It would have been much kinder to remind me how many survive.

> "You have breast cancer," said the radiation oncologist when I was agitated about drawing blood every week. I feel I am free of the disease and the radiation therapy is prevention. He could have said it differently.

plain English. When I talk about treatment, I know the physical discomfort and emotional pain the patients can experience. During chemotherapy, minutes can feel like hours. Days can feel like forever. I've been there and felt that. And I know that once you are diagnosed with cancer, there really is no end to the journey. Not a day goes by that I don't think about the disease. Nowadays, when I speak to patients, I don't just speak from things I have studied in textbooks or learned on the job. I speak from my own experience. When I talk about breast cancer, I stress the following: 1) Education about breast health should begin at an early age. 2) All women should become familiar with their breasts by performing self-exams. 3) Finding a change in your breast does not mean you have cancer. But get it checked as soon as possible. 4) If it is cancer, the sooner you find it and get treatment, the better. It might sound strange to say, but battling breast cancer has been a blessing in many ways. Today, I am a better clinical nurse specialist. It is a privilege to do work I love, with people I trust and respect, in a place that really cares about people.

(Lori Kaneshige, Honolulu, HI, diagnosed in 2002 age 34)

I had a boyfriend at the time of my diagnosis. However, I broke up with him before I started radiation treatments because our relationship was dysfunctional, and I realized life was too short to be in such relationships. I was alone since my family is all on the East Coast, and I live in California. I called my friends and family a lot though.

(Stephanie)

I've gained a lot of new friends through my experience with breast cancer. When I was diagnosed at 39, all I saw in the oncologist's office or at my radiation appointments were older women. Luckily I met a woman my age on the Web MD boards and she really helped me through chemo and radiation. She had been through it and gave me lots of tips and encouragement. When I joined the Young Survival Coalition, I met women even younger than I was who were dealing with breast cancer. Our issues were a lot different than someone who's older. I was put into menopause at a young age. I had to deal with the loss of fertility and with having no sex drive. Although I dated while going through chemo, I never told any of the men I went out with about it. I remember going out with a guy a day after a chemo treatment. He kept ordering me beers and because I didn't want to tell him I shouldn't be drinking, I just drank them. That was really stupid of me because the next day I could barely move. Not a smart thing to do when you're having chemo!

(Leslie, Springfield, VA)

I opted not to tell friends and family about my cancer, but several of my closest friends found out. I didn't want sympathy, and I didn't want them to feel uncomfortable around me. My husband had walked out on our children and me about six years before, and the few friends I still had were still dealing with that issue. I liked the anonymity of the Internet bulletin boards, although now I'd like to meet as many of these courageous women as possible. It is from them that I draw most of my strength. My friends did stick by me, but it's hard to know what to say or do if you haven't been through this.

(Rita, Santa Clarita, CA)

To imply that I never said, or thought, "Why me?" would be a lie. To sometimes want to blame myself or my husband or daughter did happen. I knew that these thoughts were not real so we talked openly about them and that helped a great deal. I do regret that we did not go to a family support group because I think this was hardest on my daughter. She was 10 at the time, and I think she has suffered more than anyone.

(Sherry Gaffney, diagnosed in 1989 at age 47)

I am a member of a group that gets together once a month and celebrates life, learn new things, talk if we need to talk, laugh all the time, and even cry if we need to cry. It's a wonderful bond, since we all understand each other in a way that those not living with cancer can't. Someone can be forgetful and say, "Oh, chemo brain," and everyone will laugh and understand. I could never say that at work, people would look at me funny.

(Julie, diagnosed at age 26)

Talk, talk, talk. I don't think my Mother ever recovered because she would never speak about it. With that said, my own daughter was 21 and did not take it well. She doesn't want to talk about it. My husband

and kids were great but a wonderful evening out with my girlfriends helped. Men cannot understand, and you don't want to worry your kids...

(pmc)

I was not sensitive to the opinions of others because I was so focused on getting good factual information. I have been very open about my illness because I see so many people who are just quivering in a heap, and I want to illustrate that there is another choice.

(Anonymous)

A male friend of mine said to me once that it really didn't matter what kind of physical scars I came away with, and that the important thing was that I survived it. I lost a couple of people I had considered my friends—the whole spectre of breast cancer raised issues for them that they couldn't deal with, and one of them told me she couldn't even see me any more without thinking about cancer.

(Dawn, Victoria, BC)

What helped me most was the support of my family and friends, doing volunteer work, and joining dragon boating. Remember these three important Es: eat sensibly, exercise regularly, enjoy life! Early diagnosis is so important. A diagnosis of breast cancer does not mean a death sentence. Do a regular monthly breast self-examination. Have a mammogram regularly.

(Liz)

Do not be afraid to let people help you. After surgery and during chemo/radiation, when people offer help, food, housecleaning, whatever, let them help you! I believe it makes others feel better too, because they tend to feel lost and helpless. Even if you don't need the house vacuumed again, let them do it! A friend sent me an uplifting note or card at least once a week throughout treatments, and it always made me smile knowing she was there and cared enough to share a little part of her day and herself with me. My husband has been amazing. It has always been "us" going through this. "We" have breast cancer, "we" are doing better, etc. He went to all appointments and the chemo treatments with me. He would have gone to radiation if they had let him in the room. I found the Young Survival Coalition, a group specifically targeting women under 40 with breast cancer. We all have similar stories and a lot to give to and receive from each other.

(Lori Hughes, diagnosed at age 35)

My partner was supportive. A part of her needed me to do things to prove that I was alive. She needed a piece of our lives to be like it was. We have a lot of wonderful friends and we historically would meet on Friday nights for a happy hour. (I never was much for the drink and especially during treatments I didn't drink.) Sometimes I went and just drank diet soda. And I would sit quietly and everybody was so kind. I would sometimes go lay in the car and from time to time one or the other of our friends would come to visit me.

(Deborah, diagnosed in 2002 at age 46)

I feel truly blessed in my life. I have had good support, a wonderful medical team and good medical coverage. There is a lot of support in my area and I am fortunate to have these things. Most of all I have a wonderful daughter who keeps me going. Family and friends are a great support. Getting out and getting involved is also helpful. Be an advocate for yourself. I did a lot of soul searching through this journey. I lost friends that I no longer needed in my life and gained friends who are needed. I met wonderful people through support groups, retreats, my church, and my involvement in "Abreast in a Boat."

(Kathy Reeve, North Vancouver, BC, diagnosed in 2000 at age 32)

Call the support lines when you need comfort. They know exactly what to say.

(L.C.)

My husband was absolutely devastated. I believe he saw himself as a widower at 42 with two small children and was terrified. He told me that he would take care of everything, kids, cooking, cleaning, bills, if I would just concentrate on getting better. Initially I felt guilty lying on the couch while he rushed around trying to keep order, but it was the best gift he could have given me. He took care of the household and took me to over 75 appointments that year. He still does all the cooking! I was always looking for a support group but felt more depressed than invigorated at the end until I came across the breast cancer survivors' dragon boat team. These women don't focus on the getting sick part as I found most support groups do, they focus on the getting well part. That's a huge difference. I have made some very good friends there.

(Catherine, Pointe Claire, QC, diagnosed in 2001 at age 39)

Paddling with the Island Breaststrokers dragon boat team was a wonderful experience for me. I would highly recommend it to any breast cancer survivor. They are a marvelous group of supportive women. They work very hard to be in shape for the many summer races they participate in. Age doesn't count. I hear there is a survivor aged 84 now paddling with them.

(Amy Murphy, diagnosed in 2002 at age 32)

Some of my girlfriends shied away from me, and that's okay, because they were thinking, "If it can happen to Becky, it can happen to me." It was just a little too close for some. We are still close, I would never lose friendship over something like that. You have to remember you're not the only one going through it. I gained new friends, and dragon boat partners, and lifelong gal pals, so even though breast cancer took something from me, I did gain something in return. I would have to say the best present I received was getting out of the hospital on my wedding anniversary and driving home in glorious sunshine listening to Jan Arden.

(Rebecca Simnor)

The one thing I really needed was to be able to talk openly. I couldn't talk about my deepest fears and problems with those closest to me. My children lived far and I didn't want to frighten them so I ended up feeling emotionally isolated. My husband was in denial. I realized that those who have not been on the cancer journey personally couldn't really understand what a loved one is experiencing while on the journey into the unknown. I realize now that it would have been much better to talk with someone, rather than trying to keep a false front. Writing in a journal was important for me, as it became the "ears" for all the things I found difficult to share with family and friends. Feeling worthy, whole and sexual despite the surgery and treatment is an important part in healing. I would recommend that women be encouraged to seek professional counseling to deal with issues of family, self-worth, and body image at the very beginning of their journey with breast cancer. Becoming a founding member of our local dragon boat team "Hope Afloat—Canada" was another positive experience. Two major side effects of breast cancer are fatigue and depression, but it has been proven time and again that there are physical, spiritual and emotional benefits from physical exercise and belonging to a team or group. The women on our team are all breast cancer survivors with a spirit of hope and courage that comes from facing challenges head on and by doing the best you can in any situation. They know from experience that there is a rich and rewarding quality of life still to be lived, filled with excitement, optimism, and camaraderie.

(Sharon Tilton Urdahl)

I am a survivor. I am the husband of a woman who died of breast cancer. My wife Carmen experienced each and every step you outline in your questionnaire. Husbands go through it all too. In my case I was with her every step of the way, 16 years worth. The cancer patient for the most part isn't able to do all of the planning and scheduling that is necessary to keep one alive.

(Frank Franco Jr.)

I joined a great support group and signed up for their program, which was my life savior. We all bonded (about 10 in each group). Lectures and swimming and exercises helped to regain my arm movement. If a friend had not recommended this, I would not have made it. We continue to meet and I have made pink "fichus" for everyone in the group. Unfortunately, we have lost a few and it saddens me.

(L.C.)

Not accepting help is either a form of denial or pride–I suffered from both.

(Debbie Garrett)

I met new people at church who had breast cancer and other types of cancer, and we were support for each other.

(Marilyn R. Prasow, Long Beach, CA, diagnosed in 2001 at age 60)

Reclaiming Life

Going on with life, moving away from illness

Still round the corner there may wait, a new road, or a secret gate.
(J.R.R. Tolkien)

My life did not turn out as planned, but it has been a good life, an unpredictable adventure in progress. Doctors healed my body as much as possible, which is their job. Healing my spirit is my own ongoing journey and an unexpected challenge, which carries hidden benefits of discovery. Two years after my treatments, I started to feel normal and excited about life again when I visited my childhood home in Finland along with my children and their partners. Changes emerge: I no longer finish reading a book if I don't enjoy it, I don't need to sew all the fabrics I bought, I can change my mind, I don't have to please others, I don't have to do everything, and I can choose what's important for me. I am slowing down on purpose and learning to live today. Increasingly I enjoy just being quiet with my own thoughts. I no longer wish to stay young but to grow old—in good health—and cherish my remaining years or decades.

And here I am, nearly five years after my cancer journey started, writing this book to celebrate life as a voice of many. One of these days I might just take a selfish sabbatical with no agenda in a cottage by the water. I would take along a few good books, my kind of music, a notebook, and some divine chocolate and coffee, and then I would watch the rain with no hurry at all.

Tips on returning to normalcy? Take your time. Rest. Rest. Exercise. Rest some more. Read. Walk. Swim. Dance. Whatever. But do eat well and rest when you need to. Go back to work when you are ready. If it is possible to work part-time and if you can afford to do so, do it.

(Maria Hindmarch)

SURVIVOR TIPS

Love yourself.
Love your body.

Go on with your life.
Move away from illness.

Don't get discouraged (I am too old, too fat, I lack energy). It might take several years to get back to your normal self after breast cancer treatments. And your new normal will be different.

Set reachable goals. Do not think that you'll run the 5 km/mile cancer marathon the first year, but you might walk it...

Whatever your age, get passionate about something new like going back to school or starting a business. Focus on your dreams again. Make more time for you.

Reorganize and simplify your life to suit your needs emotionally and physically. Reduce stress. Delete unnecessary things from your life.

I was concerned about the effect my scars from many surgeries might have on my sex life, but I have so far found those fears to be unfounded. The men in my life have made it very clear that they are pleased with the results of the reconstruction and just happy that I have had a place in their lives.

(Dawn, Victoria, BC)

The only thing I miss from pre-cancer days is my boob. I love my new life and wouldn't give it up, not even for a new boob. I have started a new business for women with mastectomies. I realized that there are only bras and bathing suits but nothing for intimacy. This is so exciting—who would have thought?

(Jacqui, Courtenay, BC, diagnosed in 2002 at age 38)

My breast that had the cancer is not the same as the other one. It is harder and quite a bit more tender. I must remind my husband of this. The disease of cancer affected me in many ways. I keep thinking about retirement, but then thought, gee, go out and enjoy yourself while you can. I wonder if I'll make it to age say, 65 or so and, if I do, what will the quality of my life be. But, then I wonder if most people 56 years old think the same thing. I would have to say that my outlook on the future is probably shorter than that of others.

(Joy McCarthy-Sessing)

Life is better. I see things differently and appreciate everything. I appreciate the little things I never noticed before. I am now taking more time for myself and getting to know myself. The difficult step for me is in finding a partner (boyfriend). Half the time I have neither the energy nor desire to pursue a relationship. I also worry about how my illness will complicate things. I miss having the energy and stamina I used to have. I miss riding my bike and hiking. I miss being able to travel freely.

(Kathy Reeve, North Vancouver, BC, diagnosed in 2002 at age 32)

As I am continually in active treatment, my life is definitely different. I have lost two breasts, good arm mobility, stamina etc. but I have gained many things also—to value each day, to do what I love and say no to the rest, to celebrate small things and drink champagne for no reason at all!

(Shelagh Coinner)

I am happy the same intimacy is still there, my husband is very supportive, and I do not feel that he sees me any differently than before my surgery. The return to work was met with tentative glances by some and outright questions by others, which I welcomed. They were sweet with flowers and cards, something I will always remember.

(Rebecca Simnor)

My life is better now but some aspects are definitely harder. It is better because my priorities are crystallized. I just don't see things the same way or get all bent out of shape about unimportant things. I don't waste my time on things that don't seem important. I have developed a number of new interests and have a wisdom I did not have before. I have much deeper spiritual beliefs and I am not afraid of death in the same way I was before. I focus more on the daily

Focus on what's good in your life. Surround yourself with positive situations. Discover reasons for gratitude.

Don't take things for granted. Ask for what you want.

Seek moments of mini-meditations. Without multitasking, fully enjoy the moments of a hot shower, hobbies, gardening, stretching, thinking, meditating, reading a good book before going to sleep.

Give your pile of breast cancer books to the hospital library, to another patient, or hide them out of sight.

Listen to your body, but do not get obsessed with cancer. Be vigilant about medical checkups for the rest of your life, even when you seem to be just fine, including mammograms and blood tests.

Don't focus on your problems all at once.

JOYS TODAY

Ordinary days.

Problem-free checkups.

Another year without
recurrence.

Feeling beloved.

Allowing others to
do things for you.

Not being perfect.

Listening to music or
rain or your thoughts.

Happy childhood
memories.

Playing with your pet.

Good sleep and beautiful
dreams.

Healing physically and
emotionally.

Seeing another sunset
and another sunrise.

gifts life offers. But, it was an incredibly painful experience to go through and I don't feel safe the way I did before. I have faced my mortality to a much greater degree, and that is a freeing and burdening experience. The treatment has affected my sex drive. I have gained weight and have gone into a much earlier perimenopause. I want to make sure my time on earth is spent doing what is important to me and giving back good things to the world.

(Lorraine Langdon-Hull)

Things are much better. I put my health ahead of everything. I made a wonderful career change and completely engaged in my new profession. In simplifying life as much as possible and only volunteering for things I fully believe in, I believe I am a better person and partner and friend.

(Anonymous)

What I miss most from my life before is a kind of innocence, the feeling of "nothing bad will happen to me." I do appreciate life more. Somehow colors are more intense. I do not postpone my plans. I do things here and now which makes life very exiting. Most of all I appreciate the people around me. I have noticed that when I give something, I get it back double.

(Katariina Rautalahti, Järvenpää, Finland, diagnosed in 1999 at age 41, recurrence in 2003 at age 45)

I will never say that I'm thankful for my cancer. In fact, I don't understand when people say that. All I know is that the past can't be undone. I can only learn from the bad experiences of life. Now, I don't put myself last. I have decided to worry about myself, to enjoy life, not to always sacrifice for the rest of the family and if they like it, fine and if they don't, tough. That is the lesson I learned but I wish I could have learned it without the cancer. I miss the years of youth I lost although each day less, as I'm getting closer to what would be a natural menopause-age. I don't fret about little things. Sweating with a hot flash does not help you feel sexy; I'd always have a fresh shower before having sex, with the window open, even in winter. I recommend brisk walks for exercise with upbeat music coming through my headset.

(Laura, Navarra, Spain, diagnosed in 1998 at age 41)

The little things don't bother me anymore, my family means more to me, and life in general is great. My family has grown closer from all that we've been through this last year. It was rough at first when they thought they were going to lose their mother. Then my last child was starting college and she didn't want to leave but we got through it. What I miss most is my sex life, it's like someone turned off the switch and it's just not working anymore. I'm just happy to be here, a year ago I never would have believed what I'd go through. How much your life can change in one year! I've signed my whole family up to do the Race & Walk for the Cure through the Susan G. Komen foundation on Mother's Day. My kids were the ones who suggested it as a present for Mom and what she's been through since last Mother's Day. I can't think of a better gift than that, can you?

(Linda Bryngelson, New Brighton, MN)

I miss the body I had before cancer.

(Dikla, North Hollywood, CA)

Eating well with good friends, laughing and enjoying togetherness.

Using your nicest tableware every day because you love it.

Strawberry ice cream when a new summer starts.

A river or ocean, water in motion, nature in all its seasons.

Allowing yourself to accept honest praise.

Being proud of yourself.

Feeling like a child again.

Starting a new project that stretches into the future.

Journaling to visit the authentic you.

Liking and loving yourself.

Grandchildren to love.

I eat better now—more fruits and vegetables even if they are not on sale. I miss the days before when I would always be thinking long term, in 15, 25 years. Now I think more about the present.

(Lorraine Zakaib, Kirkland, QC, diagnosed in 2002 at age 49)

I debated about whether or not to try to keep my online business going during this time. I did shut down briefly after my surgery to recover. My husband advised me to resume business, pacing myself so that I did not overdo it. He said that I needed something else to think about other than my cancer and the treatment. I think staying busy doing something you enjoy is important. (I could have stayed busy cleaning house, but that was not something I would have looked forward to!) It is important to keep planning ahead, to keep doing things that you enjoy.

(Debbie Garrett)

My husband and I conquered the "for better or for worse, in sickness and in health" vow. Our marriage is stronger than ever before.

(Catherine, Pointe Claire, QC, diagnosed in 2001 at age 39)

I have many concerns about my sexuality. My husband is tolerating the decrease in our sex life but once chemo is done, we'll both be interested to see if my libido returns. I miss that very, very happy feeling I had right before I was diagnosed. We were about to celebrate our 2nd anniversary. My baby was about 6 months old, which is the beginning of such a great time in his development. My job was going pretty well. Everything seemed to be so lined up and then the floor caved in. I miss the feeling that I had that maybe I had lucked out and my mother's breast cancer genes had not been passed on. What I miss most is the idea that I can carry another child.

(sams mom)

Life is better now. I take time to smell the roses as they say. I notice more of the little things that didn't seem important before my cancer. Intimacy is just as good as it was before cancer. We are planning on retiring this year. Waking up each morning beside my husband is one of the joys of life, as is seeing my kids and grandkids.

(Marianne Svihlik)

I have made a pact with myself to start exercising again. I miss my carefree attitude prior to cancer. It seems to lurk in the back of my mind. But I tend to be very optimistic. My doctors have given me a good prognosis, and I intend to do my part to make it come true.

(Rita, Santa Clarita, CA)

At one time I didn't always like the idea of another birthday, another year older. Well, now I am so happy and thankful that I am here for another birthday, another year older, aren't I lucky to be 58 now and soon 59! I enjoy family gatherings even more, so I value each one and thank God I am here to see and take part in it.

(Carole, Victoria, BC, diagnosed ate age 57)

I am more aware of my eating habits these days as I grow older. It doesn't mean I won't cheat, but I keep working at eating better. Our family is probably much closer because of this disease, more so than most families. We understand how short a life can be and appreciate knowing that we live for each day. Having to take that fancy vacation or buy all those wonderful expensive things is not a priority in our lives.

(Gwyn Ramsey)

Although cancer has ruined my life in some ways, it also has enriched it. When I have a chance to travel now, I take it. I no longer put off things that I want to do. The down side is that although I'm doing okay, I can't help but feel I'm on borrowed time and that I need to do everything I can before the cancer comes back.

(Leslie, Springfield, VA)

Better now. Cancer gave me a direction and purpose I didn't have. What I miss is my lymph nodes and arm without lymphedema! My experience had a ripple effect on my family, being particularly hard on my half-grown children. We went for counseling and found it helpful.

(Bev Parker, Naperville, IL, diagnosed in 1985 at age 40, recurrence in 2001)

Reclaiming life was and is the most difficult thing. We are never same after such an experience. It taught me a better way to view my femininity.

(Beverly Vote, Lebanon, MO, diagnosed in 2002 at age 37)

My marriage became much better, but our sex life is not as good. I am able to achieve an orgasm, but have no desire for sex.

(Anonymous)

I read articles all promising I will become noble, peaceful, a better person after cancer. Really? Where can I send such a claim? I did not see a page turn. Yet I do look at everything differently now and, when there is a problem, I calmly think that sooner or later there will be a solution and often a good one. Yet, I do realize that the small joys in my life are now the big ones, so perhaps this then is growth.

(Maarit)

Because of some of the side effects of chemotherapy, I have been unable to go back to work. I spend a lot of time at home and more time each day with my children. I worship life... I look forward to not waking up and thinking, "I have cancer." Instead, I look forward to years from now saying, "I had cancer." I was told not to eat soy, or chocolate, or drink coffee. I gave up soy, but the chocolate and coffee (I switched to decaf) won't go away.

(Dawn, North Hollywood, CA, diagnosed in 2001 at age 47)

I am a survivor! That is now my attitude. I know now that I can bounce back, that I can be productive. I am no longer so complacent about life and try to live each day to it's fullest.

(Sherry Gaffney, diagnosed in 1989 at age 47)

After a short adjustment to my new breasts, my husband and I have resumed our sexual relationship to its pre-cancer level. At first I missed my real breasts and the sensations from them but have adjusted and hardly think about it anymore.

(Helen B. Greenleaf)

Life is better in many ways... what I've learned to deal with is the scarring of my body. I don't miss anything from pre-cancer days, my life has just moved forward. I experience joys of ordinary life completely and fully. I don't dwell on being a cancer survivor, that is not who I am, since it just happens to be part of my story.

(Christine)

I feel very powerful over my own future, and very useful to others facing illness.

(Anonymous)

Since my daughter was only 6 years old when I had the recurrence and I was a business owner, I was fortunate enough to have the option to retire. As aggressive as I was in business, I pondered quite awhile on this decision. My love and concern for my family was a priority. At this point, I wonder why I pondered at all. I love being a Mommy and life is good.

(Roberta R. Nordby, Redmond, WA, diagnosed in 1984 at age 29)

I'm a survivor. Aren't we all survivors of something?

(psh)

The only thing I miss is the absence of fear of cancer. I never thought about it. My breasts were so small I never thought the cancer cells would find their way. I couldn't believe it was happening to me. I did change my diet. I take vitamins and supplements. I buy more organic products. Before I was diagnosed with cancer I seemed to put off traveling. Now I plan on traveling more. Most people think "death" when they hear the word "cancer." At first I did, too. I have talked to many people who are breast cancer survivors and who have lived for years after their diagnosis. I know of people who have died from breast cancer. I am not going to worry about it anymore. Worrying doesn't help and it is a waste of my energy. I now put my energy in my family and friends, playing piano, exercising, and reading.

(Sheryl)

My life is absolutely better now, and I would not trade my experience for anything. In a way, it was the best thing that ever happened to me. It made me realize life was too short. Moreover, it made me pursue goals I would never have otherwise pursued. I have achieved a degree. I delivered the commencement address in front of nearly 4,000 people. I had some poetry published. I'm writing a book. I'm working on a master's degree. I'm making new friends. I'm more dedicated at my job and grateful to the corporation at which I work. And I am very happy to be alive and well. Being a breast cancer survivor made my self-esteem skyrocket and made me realize there is nothing I cannot do. It is about setting goals and seizing opportunities.

(Stephanie)

Gardening and playing in the dirt is something I wait for and anticipate all winter. Do something you love, whether it is sewing, reading, catching up on some needlework or whatever. Daydream. Let your thoughts wonder. Sing. Laugh. Do whatever gives you pleasure. I don't set goals anymore. Things that once were monumental, I don't let loom over the horizon. I really look after myself, too, getting at least eight hours of sleep each night. My cancer experience has had numerous silver linings. I have met some of the most interesting, absolutely delightful people, have come to know myself and my beliefs better than I ever thought I could. I've come to value the depths of the unconditional love of my wonderful husband, who tells me every day I'm beautiful (with or without clothes on). I am pretty adamant about not having a reconstructive surgery. It's not an issue for me. I wear a prosthesis to work or to go out, otherwise my friends and family know the situation and they don't care. I find it more comfortable to be without. I've come to appreciate the wisdom, love, and support of my children. When I asked them how they got to be so wise, they said, "From you, Mom." It's OK to jump on the bed with my two-year-old granddaughter and to sing so loud the cat runs to the basement. I pamper myself and indulge in some of the most wonderful French soaps and lotions, and luxurious bed and bath linens. Expensive, yes, but I am worth it! I guess because our budget is so very tight, to the point of struggling occasionally, that it's like giving myself a hug to have these things and probably why I appreciate them so much. And every day I allow myself a treat of some sort. It may be a bowl of low-fat, sugar-free ice cream, just playing in my garden, losing myself in my latest gardening magazine. Or it may be just sitting quietly watching a simple little ladybug, a beautiful sunrise, or listening to the wind in the trees. It all brings me such pleasure. This is life! This is what it's all about. I love it! Thanks, cancer.

(Virginia, diagnosed in 2001 at age 57)

Since my cancer, I have learned not to sweat the small stuff, and I relax more. So what if the house isn't spotless? I have learned to do the things I want to do, and I have become selfish. I raised six kids. I am now 60, and this is my time.

(Chris Lengert, Campbell River, BC, diagnosed in 1996 at age 52)

My family watches me carefully. I find I am careful not to alarm them, careful of the information I give them, as the fear makes them anxious. We all have to go on living the best we can, and we can't if we're worried.

(Glennis)

We all (my family) appreciate each day, and each other so much more. We don't know when our time may run out, so we can't waste a day being mad at each other or not let each other know how much they are loved.

(Lori Hughes, diagnosed at age 35)

I think it a joy to be living here on the Victoria Island. It is such a beautiful place. I always laugh and say, "Next stop Heaven!" Not just yet though!

(Amy Murphy, diagnosed in 2002 at age 32)

I recommend kickboxing (such a feeling of power) and yoga (clears your mind, strengthens your body and puts you back in touch with your beauty, inside and out). I'm still learning how to reclaim my life. Every day is a gift.

(Alicia)

Intimacy has not changed, the love is still there, maybe even deeper as we realize how precious time is with each other. Material things are not as important as we thought they once were. I am a breast cancer survivor.

(Penny)

I feel I was robbed of a part of my youth. My life will never be the same, but it is not necessarily worse. I have learned a lot, and I have a much greater appreciation for life and love than ever before.

(Jennifer, diagnosed in 2001 at age 27)

Before cancer I was a power walker, can't do it anymore. I'm happier now, different things in my life are more important. Started singing again, became a minimalist, taking time for me. Don't know if I can be in a relationship again. I like myself.

(Cordelia Styles, Quesnel, BC)

My life is 100% better now than before cancer. I am actually living it, controlling my life, speaking up when I don't agree. I am much more active and have many more friends. I miss absolutely nothing from my pre-cancer days. There are so many joys of ordinary life... we just have to think about them.

(Joan Fox, Victoria, BC)

It has liberated me and given me greater strength and energy I didn't know I had. There is nothing like a life-threatening illness to make you examine your priorities and the meaning of your life. I am liberating myself from clutter and unnecessary stressors, doing things I've always wanted to do but put off for a better time. There is no better time, I realize now.

(Yvette, Victoria, BC, diagnosed in 2002 at age 47)

I remarried and found a wonderful friend, wife and life partner. We have been married for ten years and have two children. My new family is a constant source of joy to me, something I had once thought lost forever when my first wife died of breast cancer. As a cancer researcher myself I resolved to work on the disease and to do whatever I could to ease the suffering associated with cancer of the breast.

(Dr. Barry J. Barclay, St. Albert, AB)

My experience with cancer has brought my husband and I closer and closer. I miss my body from precancer days. I have so much numbness from surgery after the reconstruction that my body still feels alien to me. Also have numbness in my fingertips and pain in my feet from Taxol treatments. I can certainly live with this, so it's not a big deal. I'm fairly active and have a pretty healthy diet, however, I'm sure there's room for improvement. Spending time with my wonderful husband and daughter is my greatest joy here on earth. I love being a wife and mommy!

(Joni)

Cancer liberated my lifelong dream to be a writer. My children are older now, and it is my moment for glory. I continue to exercise. I had been such a stickler for eating healthy food before and ended up getting cancer anyway. I am very educated about nutrition. I am treating myself to an amazing cultural and cooking trip to Italy as my 50th birthday present to myself.

(Heather Resnick, Thornhill, ON, diagnosed in 1997 at age 43, recurrence in 1999)

I now have no sensation in my breasts whereas this used to be my pleasure zone. This has been tough for us.

(Carolyn S. Olson, diagnosed at age 37)

I have learned how to prioritize. My life is not as action-filled and can't be as exciting as it was in my 20s. But it is more focused and much more interesting now than had I not had the cancer. In December 1997, I joined a dragon boat racing team of breast cancer survivors and experienced feelings of such excitement that I hadn't had since I was a child. The team has become a "floating support group," although we are usually too excited and lively to need support. The team offers me a great combination of what I found to be my new plan, and this is my recipe for emotional and physical health—the motivation of staying physically active, the benefit of being with women who have been through it as well, and being able to speak and joke about the experience uncensored, the excitement of team sport, competition and the respect it brings from others—not pity, but respect. This team is my stability, since it gave me something to be motivated by and gave me wonderful friends and warriors in the process.

(Donna Tremblay, diagnosed in 1992 at age 33, recurrence in 1996)

I am an optimistic person, but life has always been kind of hard. I have now more confidence. Sometimes I really surprise myself with my ability to do the things I do. I am not so scared anymore. Sometimes I say when you have been able to go to work everyday with a bald head and a fire-red burnt face, there isn't anything else that seems too scary. The thing I miss from precancer is the complete and free use of my left arm. Due to the lymphedema, I have to keep it wrapped or wear a sleeve and try not to lift as much. The effect on intimacy is interesting. My partner is okay about my breasts being gone. My chest is hard though. One side is very bony and there isn't much padding. Other than that, we have improvised. Getting back to exercise was necessary. This is the key to my feeling good. I was so weak when I started but it didn't take long to build up, just a few months.

(Deborah, diagnosed in 2002 at age 46)

I definitely am convinced that my life is better now. I know myself better, I respect my body and my mind. I take more decisions than before. I make more choices. The day I was 30, I dressed in black to bury my youth. The day I was 40, I wanted to stay in bed the whole day. Now I'm just 50 and it is the first time that I am so glad that it is my birthday, even if it is my fiftieth. I live my life. I'm so glad I'm alive.

(Annemie D'haveloose, Belgium)

I sold my gallery to reduce stress and to pursue my artistic endeavors. I created "Visual Voices" (plaster casts of breast cancer patients with personal stories). I became involved with breast cancer awareness, began to speak to women's groups and write articles in the local newspapers. I organized candlelight "Celebration of Life" events and became a "visitor" support person with the Canadian Cancer Society. I arranged for interviews on our local television programming and radio stations. I became involved with our local Breast Health Group at Breast Self-Examination Clinics. I am a representative with the Alliance for Breast Cancer Information and Support B.C. & Yukon and belong to the International Support Link created during the 3rd World Conference on Breast Cancer. I found that the more positive thoughts I had, the more negative issues receded and good things seem to happen, so I became open to all possibilities. We each have gifts or lessons to receive and give and often these are recognized and brought forward during our most trying times.

(Sharon Tilton Urdahl)

I found that my first priority in life now is to enjoy it with friends.

(Sharron, diagnosed in 2002 at age 62)

Spirituality

When I do good, I feel good. When I do bad, I feel bad.
And that is my religion. (Abe Lincoln)

Spirituality was a vague concept I set aside until needed and until time allowed. Both time and need emerged with cancer, and I prayed like I meant it. Needing an anchor in my hour of need, I yearned for the innocent safety of my childhood, so I surrounded myself with guardian angels that comforted me decades ago. A friend took me to St. Joseph's Oratory in Montreal and, with a relief of hot tears, I felt a profound sense of peace envelop me to start the cancer journey. One friend lit a red candle for me whenever I had a surgery or treatment. Another friend asked for a whole congregation in a nearby church to pray for me, and I felt protected. I am not an active member of any organized religion but I do find solace in the combined philosophical wisdom of different faiths.

O Lord, help me to be pure, but not yet. (St. Augustine)

We emerged to see—once more—the stars. (Dante)

I studied Eastern and Western religions after my cancer, as well as various philosophies. I am very spiritual and utilized aspects of many religions to maintain my spirit. I believe in treating people the way you wish to be treated.

(Stephanie)

Not much change, although I more clearly understood the adage, "There are no atheists in foxholes."

(Bev Parker, Naperville, IL, diagnosed in 1985 at age 40, recurrence in 2001)

I am not a religious person, but consider myself spiritual. There is no harm or shame in receiving and sending prayers regardless of the denomination... they are all from the heart and same source and carry only positive messages of healing and love. My cousin belonged to a prayer group and had asked them to pray for me. I was very touched when I received a little white satin cloth that people I didn't even know had put their prayers into and sent to me so that I would recover my health. I pinned it into my bra so it could lie next to my breast cancer and my heart. The vision of my youngest son hiking to a mountain in Korea saying he had said prayers for me at a Buddhist temple filled me with unbelievable healing energy, courage and strength. My cousin would call me regularly and told me that every morning he went to the gym and while he exercised he said prayers for me. The night before my surgery, my close friend and spiritual leader held a First Nations "pipe ceremony" in my living room. The ceremony left me relaxed and at peace. I slept well and soundly and was ready for whatever was to unfold the next day.

(Sharon Tilton Urdahl)

I was always spiritual in the sense of appreciating nature and trying to find the good in people and being the best that I can be in my chosen path.

(Heather Resnick, Thornhill, ON, diagnosed in 1997 at age 43, recurrence in 1999)

After the diagnosis, I fell back on my religion and found comfort again in attending Sunday mass.

(Donna Tremblay, diagnosed in 1992 at age 33, recurrence in 1996)

My faith is stronger. Now I do lots of reading. A great book is *Conversations with God*. I find God in everything and joy in every aspect of life.

(Yvette, Victoria, BC, diagnosed in 2002 at age 47)

I am very grateful for what I have. Mostly I am grateful for the warm sun, the majestic mountains, the wondrous ocean, puttering around in my garden, enjoying all the flowers as they appear. This is my spirituality. I do give thanks for what I have and appreciate the comfort that my cats gave me.

(Sharron, diagnosed in 2002 at age 62)

I rediscovered my faith. I began going back to church for comfort and solace. The pastor asked if people had any joys or concerns that they would like prayer for. I stood up and told the congregation, barely getting the words out, that I had just been diagnosed with breast cancer and needed prayer. Following the service there was an outpouring of love from many women who wanted to help, a couple of whom were survivors. I felt a blanket of warmth surrounding me.

(Carolyn S. Olson, diagnosed at age 37)

I'm grateful that I've been given time to think about what has just happened in my life, both the cancer and now my husband passing on.

(Amy Murphy, diagnosed in 2002 at age 32)

I established my life as a spiritual being as best I could against the old model of me as a human being. Difficult to do since I love material things, traveling, etc. I first thought being more conscious of spiritual gifts and spiritual experiences meant giving up all earthly things and even being guilty if I enjoyed such things. I like to think that I don't have to be guilty or to feel worthy or deserving to enjoy life anew, and that material things are part of the abundance of life. The experience of breast cancer taught me that I was equating material things with love and self-worth.

(Beverly Vote, Lebanon, MO, diagnosed in 2002 at age 37)

I was thankful that my cancer had been contained in one breast, thankful that the surgery went well, thankful that follow-up tests showed no evidence of other tumors in my body, thankful that I made it through chemo and radiation with minor discomfort, and thankful that I did not wait a year to do a follow-up mammogram as recommended by the gynecologist. I am thankful that I am here today and feeling triumphant over this stage of cancer.

(Lorraine)

I became more spiritual and thank my God for giving me this additional opportunity to really experience life.

(Joan Fox, Victoria, BC)

Spiritual faith was a big part of my treatments but not something I gained from attending church. Mainly, it has been something I have revived in myself.

(Peggy Scott, Waldorf, MD, diagnosed in 2002 at age 46)

For a while there, I did question my faith, but a girlfriend that attends church regularly kept me in her prayers, and often when I need one, I'll call on her. I used to say, "Why did God give me breast cancer?" but now I believe, "He gave me the strength to get through it."

(Rebecca Simnor)

I am blessed by the knowledge of how many friends I have; I never knew or didn't open my eyes wide enough. I feel gratitude to all my doctors, nurses, technicians, family, friends, colleagues, members of my Healing Circle, and neighbors. Every little smile, bowl of soup, bag of fresh fruit, cap, card, flower was gratefully received and meant so much to me.

(Jacqui, Courtenay, BC, diagnosed in 2002 at age 38)

My Eastern Orthodox faith and my priest were one of the anchors that kept me afloat and steady as I sailed the dark and stormy cancer seas. I talked to God and the Blessed Virgin Mary a lot. I prayed and prayed and prayed only for God's will to be done and the strength to deal with whatever came my way. I also thanked God for blessing me with a close loving family, two children who would make any parents proud, and a good life.

(Helen B. Greenleaf)

I am always searching for that spiritually right place for myself. My mission has been more about accepting that this is my place. This is my spirituality. I used to search and search to get it right or to get better at it. Now, I think what works for me is that I am so grateful for my life. I also am happier to accept what is instead of always working to improve. I like life, I love to learn, but I am perhaps more at peace.

(Deborah, diagnosed in 2002 at age 46)

My church had special services for people who have had cancer.

(Marilyn R. Prasow, Long Beach CA, diagnosed in 2001 at age 60)

I have deepened and broadened my spirituality. A work in progress.

(Shelagh Coinner)

Often when I wake up in the night and the cancer thoughts start, I remind myself that my life is in God's hands. It is my responsibility to take care of myself by eating a healthy diet and exercising and getting lots of rest. Other than that it is up to God. I have really started to pray much more than I used to, and I am more open to saying prayers for others whatever their situation.

(Debbie Giroux, Langley, BC)

I have always prayed a great deal. I began to see how my prayers for others were answered during these years and beyond. The more you pray for others, the more you help yourself.

(Marie, Co. Mayo, Ireland, diagnosed in 1987, recurrence 13 years later)

I am thankful every day for my family, friends, where I live, and the beauty of nature that surrounds me.

(Penny)

I just turned to my faith in God, as I always do, to help me get through the challenges. If things did not turn out well, I would still have had my faith to get me through and to help my family and friends cope with the worst.

(Christine)

There were some dark days following my diagnosis. I hoped that the medical treatments would work but there were no guarantees. Having things to look forward to can ward off depression and self-absorption, both of which are easy to succumb to when you do not feel well. I want to sum up my personal experience with cancer with this Bible verse: "Now may the God of hope fill you with all joy and peace in believing, that you may abound in hope by the power of the Holy Spirit."— Romans 15:13.

(Debbie Garrett)

Therefore do not worry about tomorrow, for tomorrow will worry about itself. Each day has enough trouble of its own. (Matthew 6:34)

Facing Death

Regardless of prognosis, facing the possibility of dying

Good night! Good night! Parting is such sweet sorrow.
(William Shakespeare)

Facing death invaded our comfort zone. My daughter admitted later that she was afraid I'd die within two months of my diagnosis. The possibility of dying brought me profoundly interesting conversations with my children and brought me even closer to my sisters overseas. Even though it has been difficult at times, I have always loved life, curious of what more it can reveal. I don't want to die, not now when there is so much exciting life yet to live, and after wasting so much time. There is much more to learn, many enjoyable trips to take and adventures to discover. There are grandchildren not yet born to treasure. I have a big box of immortal photos to put in order and our family tree to organize, so that my children and their children will know their roots traced to many countries. And after having done all that I'd like to have still more time to do anything else I like or to do nothing at all. Cancer has made me grateful for being lucky enough to have already lived 58 good years. Accepting death as a natural part of life is a relief, but I'd like to postpone it into a distant future at my convenience and on my terms when I am really old, spent and truly ready. I wouldn't want to suffer a painful, prolonged death or to become a burden to my loved ones. I should make it easier on everyone, just in case, by putting my affairs and chaotic papers in order, but I keep postponing it into my peaceful rocking-chair era with nothing else to do. Meanwhile, I am happily busy with new projects stretching far into the future.

According to Buddhist wisdom, we learn to truly live only when death knocks at the door. Regardless of your diagnosis or prognosis, what would you do if you only had six months to live?

That it will never come again is what makes life so sweet. (Emily Dickinson)

Today is the day to live. If I only had six months to live, I would have thrown a party for all my friends, neighbors, and relatives. It would be like having my own wake and being able to enjoy it. I certainly would not request all that sad music during my funeral. That is not me, and I don't want anyone to cry just because I passed away to another world. I want a band or DJ, see people dance, laugh and having fun. I don't believe this is disrespectful for it is the way I live now. I have lived a long and good life. It has been up and down, but the trip has been great. I wouldn't change a thing.

(Gwyn Ramsey)

I gave a lot of thought to dying, what would happen to my children, whether I would die with grace and be a good role model. In my remaining time, I would get my affairs in order and spend as much time as possible with those I love best.

(Bev Parker, Naperville, IL, diagnosed in 1985 at age 40, recurrence in 2001)

Prior to my cancer diagnosis I was afraid of death. Looking at death in the face has made me less fearful. Do I want to die? No. Am I afraid of it anymore? No. I could get run over by a car tomorrow. If I knew I had only six months to live, I would ask that I not be told that. I would like to continue to hug my husband and kiss and hold my kids each and every day and night... as if it is the last time I will see them. After all, we never know when our day will come.

(Dawn, North Hollywood, CA, diagnosed in 2001 at age 47)

I thought I would kill a few people along the way but I never thought I would die.

(Mary Schmidt)

I never thought that I would die right now but I do sometimes think about dying too young. If I only had six months to live I would travel and do volunteer projects spreading joy to as many as I could in that short period of time.

(Julie, diagnosed at age 26)

Whether it is a cancer, an auto accident, flying in an airplane, crossing a busy street, etc., I do not think about death. After a serious auto accident that I was in thirty-one years ago, I decided to live life to its fullest, one day at a time. If I knew that I had six months to live, I would make sure that everyone that is important to me knows the impact that they had on my life and how much I appreciate it. I would make a video for my children telling them the joy that they brought into my life, urging them to go on with their lives and that my love for them has no bounds, not even death.

(Helen B. Greenleaf)

I am not afraid of dying. I don't look forward to the process but I'm not afraid of the afterlife. I have everything to look forward to and everything to gain. I think I would try to make the most of the time I had left without breaking the bank! I would want my family with me more and more. I would want to make things right with those I have hurt over the years and ask for forgiveness.

(psh)

Facing my fears about death was the first step in releasing me from my fears about dying. It is the most liberating feeling. While I still have emotions and fear that crop up from dying, even from a car accident or something like that, I try to quiet the fears by seeing what it is I am afraid of and why. I break it down, "If I am afraid of death, why?" Am I afraid God will send me to hell, am I afraid my husband will be sad, lonely, marry too soon, marry someone better than me, be better off, or that my kids will be depressed and won't miss me? Most fears are groundless, and fear in itself feeds fear and without breaking it down, fear will control a person's life, which means it will feed the cancer vortex, which means you keep creating more fear, instead of creating health in your life. That is the greatest peril of fear.

(Beverly Vote, Lebanon, MO, diagnosed in 2002 at age 37)

If I knew I had only six months to live I would travel like crazy to all the places I've always wanted to go to and do the things on my "things to do before I die" list. The truth is that I would probably spend my time in treatment, even experimental treatments.

(Joy McCarthy-Sessing)

My partner was afraid I'll die but I knew I won't die overnight from this. If I had six months to live, I might do something stupid like my friend did. She cleaned her house and threw away all her old underwear before surgery, but she survived and regretted, because it was perfectly good underwear after all. Or I might clean my papers. I wish I would do something wonderful instead, travel perhaps to New Zealand, cook good food and invite all my friends.

(Maarit)

I never felt I'd die; I felt it was a sign to get involved to help eradicate this disease.

(Deb Haggerty, diagnosed at age 51)

We all will die. But will we all really live in the time allotted to us? If I knew I had six months... I would travel with my family and waste a lot of money leaving them with some great memories.

(Anonymous)

I thought I might die. Even going under anesthesia twice was a fear. I told my family not to be sad for me if the worst happened, because I felt my life has already been so full, and I've been blessed beyond what I ever expected. This has been a time of renewal with relatives and friends telling me how much they care. Many sincere "I love yous" have been said.

(Diane Dorman)

Somehow it is very strange that it seems like only cancer patients are expected to fear death and think about death. What about other people? Do they live forever? Other people die as well. It is not a big difference; everybody dies after all and nobody knows when.

(Katariina Rautalahti, Järvenpää, Finland, diagnosed in 1999 at age 41)

I am a real pack rat. If I had only six months to live I would clean out my house. At one time I thought that I would be lying in my bed and my friends would come to visit me and so I purchased $600 worth of bedding. Now it is all worn out, and I don't worry about it.

(Esther Matsubuchi, North Vancouver, BC)

I did think I might die. It scared the hell out of me, but the whole experience made me know that we are truly more than our physical bodies, and that death is a transition to something else. I am not so scared of death anymore, and I believe there are other dimensions of reality beyond the physical. In this sense, it was truly an amazing experience.

(Lorraine Langdon-Hull)

I know I will die as my disease is advanced. But for now I am well and continue to focus on my many blessings. I would like to learn to live each day with purpose and passion.

(Shelagh Coinner)

If I knew I had six months to live, I'd want to live it. I'd want to visit people I hadn't seen for a long time and do things with the young people in my life.

(Cheryl Otting, Elkford, BC, diagnosed at age 2002 at age 53)

My house is in order and I cannot do anything... I am in God's presence every moment.

(L.C.)

I have decided that it is not important how long I live but how much I enjoy my life. I am much more afraid of being disfigured or disabled or debilitated.

(Anonymous)

I saw my life that I hadn't lived yet literally flash before my eyes. Then I told myself that I had to beat it, because my husband and sons would not be able to handle life without me, and that was that. I would spend time writing some letters for the future to help my children go through important events in their future knowing I was still with them in spirit.

(Christine)

Sure, I'm going to die, I just don't know when and don't think about it. This isn't something that we cancer survivors think about, ever. We are survivors, not dwellers.

(Jacqui, Courtenay, BC, diagnosed in 2002 at age 38)

I still feel very vulnerable and believe I might not conquer this disease. Some days I feel strong and other days (especially when I hear someone has died from breast cancer) I think it could be me next. Not a day passes by that I don't have a mini panic attack, especially at night. But it passes and I wake up again the next day and I think, "I've been given one more day."

(Catherine, Pointe Claire, QC, diagnosed in 2001 at age 39)

I still feel like I will die from this disease, even though all reports are fine right now. It is not something that I dwell on, and I don't feel like I am being pessimistic but realistic. We are all terminal, when you get down to it. It is just that some of us have had to face our mortality sooner than others do.

(Peggy Scott, Waldorf MD, diagnosed in 2002 at age 46)

My priorities now have changed. I try to look at other people and consider that they might be going through something like I did. I still had to go to the grocery store, and I'd see dozens of people every day that had no idea I was facing my mortality. I try to keep these things in perspective. I'm not always successful, but I'm much more aware of what is important to me.

(Julie Austin, Little Rock, AR, diagnosed in 2000 at age 30)

The thought of dying is always in the back of my mind. If I do end up dying as a result of my cancer, at least I will feel that I did everything I could to make myself healthy. If I knew I had a short time to live, I would try to take a trip to somewhere I always wanted to go with my kids. I would spend as much time with them as possible and try to help them understand that I will love them forever. I want to live my life to the fullest to show them that there is life after cancer. But they know also that if I should die from this that I'm OK with it.

(Rita, Santa Clarita, CA)

Successful pain management is a very important issue that greatly affects quality of life, especially in advanced cases.

(Dr. Barry J. Barclay, St. Albert, AB, lost his wife to breast cancer)

My six months would be filled with living, learning and loving.

(Heather Resnick, Thornhill, ON, diagnosed in 1997 at age 43)

If I knew I only had six months to live... I'd visit or write to all the people in my life to let them know what I appreciate about them, the gifts I see in them to share with the world, how they have touched my life, and to encourage them in the future. Maybe we should always be focused on these things anyway, whether we have six months to live or 80 years.

(Joni)

You come to realize just how short life is and that you really have no time to waste. You need to have fun every day. Enjoy life as much as you can.

(Jennifer, diagnosed in 2001 at age 27)

When I first heard the word cancer, I was physically sick and scared. For a few days, everything was a blur. My doctor told me not to look ahead but just go through each step. It worked.

(Cordelia Styles, Quesnel, BC)

If I only had six months to live... Certainly a trip to foreign countries or around the world might be nice, but I think I would spend that time just living each day, each moment, with every breath I had, caring about what is important to me and my family. Worrying what the world thinks just doesn't matter. I guess you could say I've developed an attitude!

(Virginia, diagnosed in 2001 at age 57)

I found the thought of dying very frightening. It made me think of my mom and dad a lot.

(Carole, Victoria, BC, diagnosed at age 57)

Yes, I thought I might die if the cancer spread to other organs. I still wanted to fight it as best I could. If I had but 6 months to live then I know for certain that I would take the trips to see my children and grandchildren in their homes. That would make me very happy.

(Amy Murphy, diagnosed in 2002 at age 32)

---

196 • Facing death

I know that my time on earth is limited. I make more decisions on my own. I make more choices. I know better what I want. If I had six months left, I would travel to the six continents and enjoy nature and the people.

(Annemie D'haveloose, Belgium)

The thought of it is incomprehensible to me.

(Rebecca Simnor)

My doctor said it well, "You must face your own death and come to terms with it." Death is inevitable, and everyone must part eventually. I am not afraid to die, but I intend to stay around for a long time to come.

(Yvette, Victoria, BC, diagnosed in 2002 at age 47)

Make a list of things you want to do and do them. Throw or give away everything you don't need. Simplify. Say "I love you." Live.

(Alicia)

I never thought I would die but I did examine death, and it helped me reorder my priorities to accomplish more important things for the rest of my life.

(Anonymous)

I thought I might die but I dismissed it the following day after talking to my mentor (also a survivor). A positive attitude and faith is what we need to carry us through the ordeal.

(Stephanie)

I was afraid. I was afraid of leaving those I loved, afraid of suffering in a hospital bed or being "out of it" if I was drugged for pain, and afraid of having those I loved have to "watch me die" little by little which, to me, is a senseless suffering. I didn't and don't want them to go through that.

(Laura, Navarra, Spain, diagnosed in 1998 at age 41)

Humor

Laughter, the proverbial best medicine

It's not that I'm afraid to die, I just don't want to be there when it happens. (Woody Allen)

"I am a licensed professional cancer," wrote Deborah accidentally in her entry for this book. Puzzled, I was wondering if I was missing her point since English is not my mother tongue until she explained she meant to write that she is a licensed professional counselor. Humor, sometimes silly or unintentional and sometimes dark, finds its way even into cancer and gives a welcome relief.

My daughter made me a healthy get-well meal days after my diagnosis so I exclaimed, "This is the best meal ever, and I'll never forget it for as long as I live... which might not be that long...," and we cried and we laughed and then we ate heartily. One day, I went to my favorite grocery store, and the cashier innocently greeted everyone, "Good morning and how are you?"— so when it was my turn, I blurted out without thinking, "Very bad, I have cancer." I did not mean to be funny, but later I was talking about it to a friend who had also recovered from cancer, and we laughed hysterically and it felt great. At first I didn't want to waste my remaining days on earthly tasks and pleasures. Soon, however, the dirty dishes piled up and I just had to see who was on Larry King Live, plus I missed my morning paper with a good cup of coffee, so I promptly resumed my routine, whether I lived or died.

When angry, count four; when very angry, swear. (Mark Twain)

I find my life rather funny today. I get up in the morning and say out loud to myself, "Now where did I lay my breast?" I couldn't say that before.

(S.R., Columbus, OH)

I would have lost my sanity without humor. I began wearing a wig when my daughter was around two. Instead of saying she wanted to go somewhere, she'd say, "Mommy, put your hair on." She knew we weren't going anywhere without that hair.

(Julie Austin, Little Rock, AR, diagnosed in 2000 at age 30)

I made it a point to tell my friends to make me laugh, and they did. Some days I felt worse than other days, and I am sure I did not smile as easily on those days.

(Peggy Scott, Waldorf, MD, diagnosed in 2002 at age 46)

It really helps to have a sense of humor. I have never laughed as much or enjoyed life more. I have learned not to take crap from anyone.

(Chris Lengert, Campbell River, BC, diagnosed in 1996 at age 52)

My sister and I had cancer at the same time and we each bought a wig. She named her wig "Brown Betty." Instead of asking her hubby if her wig looked presentable, she would ask if Betty looked okay.

(Kristina, diagnosed in 1995 at age 39)

I did not lose my sense of humor during cancer; if you lose this, you are already dead.

(Karen Lisa Hilsted, Denmark)

I did not lose my sense of humor—I fell back on it. I was always kind of a prude, very shy about my body. In radiation I had to undress from the waist up and put on a hospital gown, then walk across the room. I was horrified at first because people in the waiting room could see me. After my 11th treatment, I was so tired and had become so used to the gown and the hallway cross, that I was walking out of the waiting room when one of the technicians called me back, "Donna, where are you going?" "Home," I said, confused at the question. Until she answered, "Dressed like that?" I looked down and I was still in the hospital gown! We laughed so much and so did people in the waiting room. The technician said, "I was tempted to follow you to see how far you were going to go before you noticed!"

(Donna Tremblay, diagnosed in 1992 at age 33, recurrence in 1996)

"Don't take life too seriously. You'll never get out of it alive!" This is one of the best slogans I ever heard. When all my hair had fallen out, I took some pictures with a boy who shaves all his hair on purpose. Two bald laughing heads! It was fun and I still like to look at those pictures from time to time.

(Annemie D'haveloose, Belgium)

I call myself "Uni-boob." One day I was teaching a class when my falsie slipped out of my bra and lodged in the waistband, so I kept talking with my arms glued to my side while backing out of the door.

(Yvette, Victoria, BC, diagnosed in 2002 at age 47)

I tried not to lose my wit during my journey. At a Tai-Chi class, my body was contorted in many directions. Ooops, my prosthesis was up around the top of my shoulder somewhere. I made a comment about it taking talent to be able to do that with one's breast and put it back in place. Everyone laughed. It eased a moment that could have become embarrassing.

(Virginia, diagnosed in 2001 at age 57)

At work, when I'm trying to persuade someone to see things my way or give me more money for a program I wish to pursue, sometimes with colleagues I'm close to I say, "Don't make me use that cancer card!'

(sams mom)

When you can laugh again, you are reaching a stage of knowing that healing is available. Humor is not only a powerful healing tool, it is the signal that you are heading in the right direction. Laughter has power over fear—deep belly laughing, not stifled laughter trying to cover our pain or fear, but deep soul laughter. It stirs within us the reminder that living life, not just being a puppet existing but feeling life and letting it vibrate within our body, our emotions, and within our soul is a deeply liberating experience. Laughter and humor raises us from being victims to new perspective of feeling. It helps remind us to feel differently than what cancer would want us to feel.

(Beverly Vote, Lebanon, MO, diagnosed in 2002 at age 37)

My cancer journey is ongoing so I try to laugh as much and as often as I can, even if it hurts.

(Shelagh Coinner)

Laughing at my bald head, laughing about the expression on a young boy's face when he came to my door and saw me hairless. Talking rudely with my breast cancer volunteer and laughing uncontrollably with her. I don't think I lost my sense of humor, I think I gained it.

(Cheryl Otting, Elkford, BC, diagnosed in 2002 at age 53)

My coworkers played a game called "Spotting Dawn" because I had a number of different wigs in various styles and colors.

(Dawn, Victoria, BC)

There is perhaps no greater ability one can possess than to laugh at oneself.

(Stephanie)

Our small son had lost all of his hair (from chemo due to leukemia) and today he can relate to my husband who is bald. We all laugh about that. No, I didn't lose my sense of humor during treatments, just my energy.

(Gwyn Ramsey)

I wanted to get a T-shirt that said "chemo sucks" and wear it to my treatment, but I was afraid that some older people might think that it wasn't funny at all so I didn't. A lot of older patients are more serious about this than the younger crew. I'm not sure why that is since they have lived most of their lives already.

(Jacqui, Courtenay, BC, diagnosed in 2002 at age 38)

I wore a wig for a few months. I usually took it off before I left the office and donned my cap for my drive home. One day, being in a hurry, I didn't take the wig off until I was pulling out of the parking lot. As I whipped it off my head and threw it on the back seat, another car passed by and I couldn't help but notice the startled look on the other driver as the wig went flying into the backseat!

(Christine)

I am not inhibited anymore. I always say what's on my mind. I really don't care what people think of me so I dance in the middle of the street if I want to.

(Catherine, Pointe Claire, QC, diagnosed in 2001 at age 39)

My son has a great sense of humor and it has been a huge blessing. When I email him I sign myself "Baldy." My parents took me to a chemo treatment once. My mother came into the room to see what all the laughing was about because she could hear my laughter in the waiting room. And there's plenty to laugh about. I make a truly ugly bald person, and I laugh when I see myself in the mirror, partly because I'd probably cry if I didn't.

(Rita, Santa Clarita, CA)

Humor is important and has always kept me going. Laughing about breast cancer with those "in the boat" is fun and gives us a special connection.

(Bev Parker, Naperville, IL, diagnosed in 1985 at age 40, recurrence in 2001)

The whole cancer journey started with misunderstanding when my doctor called after biopsy to say, "I am sorry but the sample doesn't look good." I was just leaving for a European business trip so in rush I assumed he was my business contact. I angrily argued that nothing can be wrong with the samples, since I had checked them myself! One elderly man at the hospital was worried that if I lose my breast it would devastate my husband since I am so young and beautiful. I was wondering who would take my cancer but there were not bad enough enemies. I was even ready to trade my life with a bum on the street corner to sell shoelaces for a daily "Cambina." I didn't stop to think what illnesses the poor bum had and felt guilty about my imaginary trade later.

(Maarit)

Through laughter, my tears have found another place to call home. I think that tears of joy, or tears of sadness, live together to get anyone through a rough time. Everyday that I wake up with the grass under my feet is a good day. When I wake up and the grass is above me, I have big problems.

(Dawn, North Hollywood, CA, diagnosed in 2001 at age 47)

I didn't lose my sense of humor during treatment, but it probably was stuffed in a closet for awhile.

(Sheryl)

This is not a funny thing but I meet people who tell me how their diagnosis were missed, and we can laugh at it now that we are recovered.

(Esther Matsubuchi, North Vancouver, BC)

No, one can never lose their sense of humor. It is the one thing that will always be there to help you out. Just about all caregivers, friends, relatives, neighbors, react favorably to humor, especially to humor about oneself.

(Joy McCarthy-Sessing)

The plastic surgeon was quite good looking. When he said to let my stomach out so that he could make sure there was enough stomach fat needed to reconstruct a new breast, I didn't want to let him know I had a stomach that big. Finally, after he convinced me to quit holding my breath, my husband suggested that he roll me over and take some off the backside instead. Men! Further to this, when I got the nipple reconstructed at a later date, he pierced my belly button at the same time! Fancy that...

(Marylynn)

My humor helped others feel at ease around me.

(Lori Hughes, diagnosed at age 35)

My husband has a goofy sense of humor and at times I didn't appreciate it when I was going through treatments. I think I can laugh with him better now than I used to. My 2-year-old daughter can be very silly and is developing a fun sense of humor. I often laugh out loud with her, and I know this is a great gift.

(Joni)

I found that I was almost never laughing. That's why I really appreciated when I'd hear a joke from someone.

(Laura, Navarra, Spain, diagnosed in 1998 at age 41)

For years, after getting out of a shower, I would complain to my husband about the two small extra "breasts" I had on either side of my tummy which were due to a caesarean section. After I decided on the double mastectomy, I told my husband that the two on top are being vacated and the two below were "moving on up."

(Helen B. Greenleaf)

Humor is important, but I have found that it is easiest to laugh with the members of my support group. It helps.

(Katariina Rautalahti, Järvenpää, Finland, diagnosed in 1999 at age 41)

Let loose and laugh about treatments, side effects, whatever, and I guarantee you'll feel better.

(Anonymous)

Just before the mammotome biopsy, I asked the radiologist, "Since we are suctioning out breast tissue, would you mind doing the thighs, stomach and buns also?" The room liked that.

(Toni)

I didn't pay much attention to underwear choice as I figured I would be in my birthday suit as before. When the nurse said take everything off but my underwear, I looked down to see my leopard print french cut bikinis.

(Diane Dorman)

You have to laugh or you will cry. It is part of being fearless.

(Anonymous)

I'm one of those people who don't get jokes, but my friends and I usually find things to laugh about. This didn't stop because of cancer.

(Maria Hindmarch)

We were once caught while I was giving my wife a morphine shot in the backside in a storage room of a local restaurant. It appeared that we were in the middle of some kind of unusual sexual practice.

(Dr. Barry J. Barclay)

I never lost my sense of humor and my husband always had his. He had to hold my drain while I showered the first time after surgery and got completely soaked fully clothed.

(Penny)

Because of my dad, our family knew a lot of the medical people helping me. My radiologist went to medical school with my brother and she was about my age. She went on vacation during my treatment and one of her partners filled in. So I'm lying on the slab waiting to be nuked, stripped to the waist. Suddenly, this handsome head of brown hair comes into my vision and he says, "Hi, I'm Dr. So-and-so and I lived with your brother during med school." So I said, "That means we were at the same parties together. Why don't you just give me a pelvic and I'll really have nothing to hide from you!" I thought he was going to die laughing. When I got cancer, I thought that it couldn't be real because Barbie never got cancer. They have an Astronaut Barbie, a Doctor Barbie, a Teacher Barbie, but there's no Breast Cancer Barbie. So I made one. My girlfriends came over one afternoon and we defaced Barbie. It was hell cutting through those plastic boobs with a paring knife. I still have her, but very few people see the humor in this as much as I do.

(Mary Schmidt)

Driving along Boulevard René-Lévesque in Montreal on a beautiful sunny summer day with a friend in her convertible car with the top down and my hair falling out and flying through the air. Imagining my hair sticking to the windshields of the cars behind us!

(Lorraine Zakaib, Kirkland, QC, diagnosed in 2002 at age 49)

At the entrance to the hospital I felt as if I had made a deliberate decision to check my brain at the door and let everyone else do the thinking for me. The ultrasound technician said, "This screen shows me that all your body parts are where they are supposed to be and they are working well." We both laughed, and this was my first experience with the power of comic relief.

(Vivia Chow)

I had visions of delivering my home-business humor speeches that fall either half-bald or in an ill-fitting wig, which unsettled me far more than the thought of losing a breast.

(Barbara Brabec)

The whole procedure was surreal. The surgeon, the radiologist, the entire world looking at my breast! The only thing I could do was laugh about it because if I didn't I couldn't get through it. I didn't lose my breast. But if the cancer comes back, I'll whack it off so fast it'll make your head spin.

(Mary Schmidt)

Quit worrying about your health; it will go away.
(Robert Orben)

If you are going through hell, keep going.
(Winston Churchill)

A hospital is no place to be sick.
(Samuel Goldwyn)

Afterthoughts

More insight from survivors

The question is not whether we will die, but how we will live.
(Joan Borysenko)

I asked "Anything else?" at the end of my questionnaire for this book in case I had forgotten something important. These are some of the gems I received.

Writing about my experience with breast cancer has felt good. It's like digging in warm soil in the spring with my hands. Thank you! God's blessings to you.

(Sheryl)

I would never ask to be part of this "club" that I found myself in... but what I am proud of is knowing that I am part of a group of women who show courage, great fortitude and a sense of humor... women who can love and care for others... women who have learned life's greatest lesson that it doesn't matter what you do to earn a living, it's how you treat people and what you do to earn the respect, love and caring of others. This is what really matters.

(Christine)

It's just a hard thing. Use your resources. Your best friend in this can be yourself. While parts of your body may self-destruct, there are other parts that can never be taken away, the essence of who we are. My body has changed, but if anything, I am stronger. I won't even pretend that I am grateful for the experience but the experience is real, and I am going to take from it everything I can. It has offered me a wealth of stories, food for the imagination, and it has allowed me to know strength that I would never have known I had.

(Deborah, diagnosed in 2002 at age 46)

It is so important to surround yourself with positive people. Stay clear of those that have terrible stories to tell, they are not you. I remember the first person I told after being diagnosed, not because she was my best friend, but because I knew she'd say, "So? We ran a marathon together, this will be a piece of cake", and she did say just that. My best friend would have cried, and I did not need that at that moment; we did that later.

(Rebecca Simnor)

One of the most important things for me to know was that women could live more than a few years after a diagnosis of breast cancer. I was enjoying a cup of coffee with a friend when a beautiful, poised older woman sitting at the next table interrupted our conversation. She had been diagnosed 40 years earlier with breast cancer and was now celebrating her 75th birthday. I have since met women who have been diagnosed over 20 and 30 years ago. By sharing their stories they give hope and inspiration to others. Ask for what you need physically, mentally and spiritually from your physician, family and friends. And if you can, try to share your thoughts with them as they are on the journey with you and most likely want to help but may feel helpless. Make certain that your young children and teens are given counselling so that they have support and guidance to help them deal with what is happening with you and to them... Keep your focus on healing. One of my most favorite sayings is: "While the sick man has life, there is hope..." (Cicero 43 B.C.) I have learned that time is a gift that I cannot hold or keep so I'm grateful for any additional days I have been given. Having faced death, I realize living is not about having or not having "things"— it's the actual journey and the people on it that give me the richness of life. I have a life rich with a variety of experiences. Five years after the diagnosis, I held my first precious grandchild in my arms after thinking I may not live long enough to do so.

(Sharon Tilton Urdahl)

Whenever my children used to complain about a big school project, or other large task or seemingly unattainable result, I would ask them, "How do you eat an elephant?" And they would answer, "One bite at a time." I dealt with the cancer elephant one step at a time. Each step was the size that I knew I could handle at that particular time. Consequently, some, such as coming to grips with the diagnosis, were tiny baby steps taken slowly. Others were huge and faster such as scheduling appointments, setting up and getting what was needed for my complementary therapy regime. I believe that one can be and stay positive when you feel that you have at least some control in what is happening in you life. So, it is up to you to take control of all that you can, physically and emotionally, and then tackle that elephant, one step at a time.

(Helen B. Greenleaf)

When I reached my 5-year anniversary from cancer, I held an "Earth Angels" party for about 80 guests. They had done so much for me and it was a pleasure to give something back. I chose a popular restaurant and decorated the room with pink balloons and with pink roses in table vases. The guests were required to wear their wings, no matter what type. I wrote a speech to thank everyone for all that they had done. It was a wonderful event. If it weren't for all the prayers and good wishes and positive attitudes from this group of people, my healing time would have been longer. I love all the people that were there that day. They are very special to me, and I will always remember their kindness, concern and prayers.

(Kristina, diagnosed in 1995 at age 39)

It was real nice during my journey when friends would just call to talk about ordinary life and not about my cancer.

(Carolyn S. Olson, diagnosed at age 37)

I climbed the Aconcagua, 6959 meters (www.BeyondTheWhiteGuard.org about seven women with breast cancer climbing Mount Aconcagua). During our climb we often talked about how we would feel if we didn't get to the top. Everybody said they would not be disappointed. I did not say anything, as I knew within myself that I had to get to the summit. When the team left base camp and I was left behind due to a severe stomach infection, I knew I was going to join them even though everybody told me stomach infections and summits do not go well together. 24 hours later with 6 litres (quarts) of muddy boiled water, 2 cokes and antibiotics, I packed my things at 6 AM, joined a carrier who was going up and met my team for a breakfast at Camp Canada, 4800 meters. From there we went on to Camp Nido de Condores at 5300 meters. I was well again. You see, cancer, chemo and stomach infections cannot beat me! When I got to the summit, I was pleased and felt, "Let's get the pictures taken and get down!" I was very excited about getting to the top; the climb up is hard but the climb down (3 days) is just as hard. You have not finished before you are standing in the shower 14 days after you were there last.

(Karen Lisa Hilsted, Denmark)

Even though it was the worst thing that could happen, positive things came out of it. I learned about love and friendship and family. I love my family, friends, doctors, breast cancer support group and church.

(Cordelia Styles, Quesnel, BC)

Always remember, where there is life, there is hope! My father always said, "Yesterday is gone, forget it. Today is here, live it. Tomorrow may never come." (Jack Caslin) In my worst moments, I always remembered that and tried to live today. And I remembered that there were wonderful friends and family in heaven watching over me and that if I died, they would be there for me.

(Marie, Co. Mayo, Ireland, diagnosed in 1987, recurrence 13 years later)

Watch your weight. Exercise, walk, whatever, with upbeat music to lift the spirit. There's nothing wrong with having a good cry in the bathtub once in awhile. You release tension. Then go out and treat yourself to some chocolate, a coffee, whatever. Dancing alone in the house to loud upbeat music helps when you start to feel sad.

(Laura, Navarra, Spain, diagnosed in 1998 at age 41

Live for today, smile a lot and remember. . . when the sun comes up, you can do anything. We all have choices and decisions to make so make them wisely, and enjoy every moment you have. Life is wonderful.

(Gwyn Ramsey)

It was a good experience for me but I don't care to go through it ever again!

(psh)

After a while it becomes difficult for people to keep hearing the same fears but sometimes we need to keep voicing them. After writing all this down, I can see I am moving on somewhat, which is encouraging.

(Catherine, Pointe Claire, QC, diagnosed in 2001 at age 39)

Breast cancer isn't a death sentence, and whatever changes you have to make, make the most of them. Take advantage of the good things and get rid of the bad things. I love my life and enjoy everything that it has to offer, even the jerk that just cut me off.

(Jacqui, Courtenay, BC, diagnosed in 2002 at age 38)

Thank you for letting me tell my story. I found it to be a very cathartic experience. I hope others will find hope and strength in the pages of your book. Thanks for the opportunity to share.

(Rita, Santa Clarita, CA)

Writing this brought back many memories and tears. Hopefully some of my comments will help others.

(Sharron, diagnosed in 2002 at age 62)

Blessings to the caregivers of the world! Without them, a breast cancer patient cannot survive. Being a caregiver unto ourselves is very, very important to remember. Nurture your emotions of self-worth, and don't let fears run your life. Let love be your steering mechanism. What we feel is what we are. When you feel sick, remember that by getting quiet and even meditating you can pretend to feel well. It is in the feeling that our cells pay attention. Feel yourself powerful and strong and courageous. Feel yourself well, in the small moments. As you lay down to sleep, imagine yourself feeling better the next morning. Blessings to the caregivers, may we each be one.

(Beverly Vote, Lebanon, MO, diagnosed in 2002 at age 37)

Thank you for giving me the chance to go back along my journey... I haven't done that for a long time. I'm absolutely positive my life is better now. I only have good dragons now.

(Joan Fox, Victoria, BC)

Doctors need more training in how to deal compassionately with patients and if they can't, at least have a nurse present at the start when the diagnosis is given. Nasty, bitter secretaries should be replaced or transferred. Oncology department should be decorated, light and happy; we're not all dying! Diagnosis should not be given over the phone. More information and guidance should be offered about going back to work.

(Lorraine Zakaib, Kirkland, QC, diagnosed in 2002 at age 49)

Breast cancer wellness has come a very long way but unfortunately has a long way to go. I was petrified to have to wait a week for the biopsy results. It is a cruel and unusual punishment. If I could change things at this moment for women, it would be from start to finish of these first moments of terror to move expeditiously. Don't make the patient wait for the biopsy, biopsy results, and further surgery if necessary. It takes 10 years off your life waiting and not just yours.

(Toni)

I feel richer for having gone through these illnesses. I am usually the one that takes care of others; they now know that I am only human and can get ill also. I know how I react to being ill, and I know how lucky I am to have so many wonderful friends and family.

(S.R., Columbus, OH

One day maybe we won't know anyone who's getting diagnosed with breast cancer as maybe it'll be gone from this world. Wouldn't that be nice?

(Cheryl Otting, Elkford, BC, diagnosed in 2002 at age 53)

Thanks for doing this book to help others with breast cancer. It was therapeutic for me just to write about this.

(Joni)

Spend the afternoon, you can't take it with you.
(Annie Dillard)

There is more to life than increasing its speed. (Mohandas Gandhi)

Glossary

Antidepressants: Drugs used to treat or alleviate depression

Aspirate: To insert a fine needle into a tissue to draw out fluid or tissue.

Axilla: Armpit.

Axillary lymph nodes: Lymph nodes found in the armpit.

Axillary node dissection: Surgical removal of the lymph nodes found in the armpit region.

Benign: Not cancerous.

Bilateral prophylactic mastectomy: Both breasts are surgically removed to potentially prevent breast cancer in high-risk cases.

Biopsy: Removal of a sample of tissue or cells (to see if cancer is present).

Calcifications: Small calcium deposits in breast tissue that are detected by mammography. They can occur with breast cancer but also in benign breast tissue.

Cancer: Disease of abnormal, uncontrolled growth of cells.

Cellulitis: Skin infection caused by bacteria.

Chemotherapy: The use of chemicals to treat cancer.

Clean or clear margins: The edge of tissue that surrounds the removed tumor and is free of cancer.

Core biopsy: With a needle, a small portion is removed from a lump without surgery.

Cyst: Buildup of normal fibrous tissue.

Dorsi flap (latissimus muscle flap): Reconstruction after mastectomy or partial mastectomy by transferring a flap of skin and muscle taken from back to create a new breast.

DCIS: (Ductal carcinoma in situ) The cancer at the earliest stage. This type of breast cancer is confined only to the ducts of the breast.

Ducts: Channels that carry body fluids. Breast ducts transport milk from the breast's lobules to the nipple.

Excisional biopsy: Taking a whole lump out surgically.

Expander: Used in saline breast implant, a hollow, empty sack is placed behind the muscle, and gradually injected with saline to stretch the skin out.

Fibroadenoma: Benign fibrous tumor of the breast.

Frozen shoulder: Painful stiffness of the shoulder that makes it hard to lift the arm over your head.

Hormone receptor test: Test to determine whether or not a tumor is hormone dependant.

Hot flashes: A symptom of menopause, sometimes brought on by antihormone treatments, characterized by sudden feelings of intense heat, blushing, or sweating, starting at face and neck.

HRT: Hormone replacement therapy. Hormone-containing medications taken to offset the symptoms and other effects of the hormone loss that accompanies menopause.

Implant: An artificial breast made of saline (saltwater) or silicone by a plastic surgeon.

In situ: Confined to the site of origin. Cancer has not invaded the surrounding tissue beyond its site of origin.

Incisional biopsy: Taking a piece of the lump out to test for malignancy.

Infiltrating cancer: Invasive cancer which has spread to nearby tissue, lymph nodes under the arm, or other parts of the body beyond its site of origin.

Inflammatory breast cancer: Rare form of breast cancer. The skin may appear red, swollen, warm, and might be mistaken for an infection.

Invasive breast cancer: Cancer that has spread beyond its site of origin. Same as infiltrating cancer.

Local recurrence: A second tumor at the same site from which the original has been removed.

Lumpectomy: Surgery to remove a lump and a small margin of healthy tissue surrounding it but without removing the entire breast.

Lymphatic system: The tissues and organs that produce, store, and transport cells that fight infection and disease.

Lymph nodes: Small glands located throughout the body that filter and destroy bacteria.

Lymphedema: Accumulation of lymph fluid in the tissue under the skin due to damaged or missing lymphatic vessels or nodes. The accumulation of fluid creates excessive swelling.

Malignant: Cancerous.

Mammogram: An X-ray of the breast.

Margins, clean or clear: The edge of tissue that surrounds the removed tumor and is free of cancer.

Markers (ink): Used to guide radiation marks; will gradually disappear.

Mastectomy: Surgery to remove the breast.

Metastasis: Spread of cancer to other parts of the body, usually through lymphatic vessels or bloodstream.

Microcalcification: Tiny calcifications in the breast tissue detected usually by a mammogram. If clustered, they can signal a ductal carcinoma in situ.

Mouth sores: Destruction of cells in the mouth, caused sometimes by chemotherapy drugs in the treatment of breast cancer.

Node negative: Cancer has not spread to the lymph nodes.

Oncologist: Physician who specializes in the treatment of cancer.

Oophorectomy: Removal of ovaries.

Palpating: Pressing the breast surface with fingers to detect lumps.

Pathology report: Analysis of the biopsy, includes the diagnosis and description of the disease.

Port-a-cath (or Hickman): A catheter device that is surgically placed under the skin and into a major blood vessel, used to draw blood or to give chemotherapy drugs.

Prognosis: Likely outcome of disease in a patient.

Prosthesis: Artificial replacement of removed body part; in breast cancer, a removable replacement for a missing breast.

Protocol: Predetermined treatment plan for groups with similar medical conditions. Usually used when referring to treatment with experimental drugs.

Radiation therapy: The use of high-dose X-rays to treat cancer.

Radiologist: Physician trained in performing X-ray procedures and reading X-rays.

Reconstruction: In breast cancer, artificial breast created by plastic surgeon after mastectomy.

Recurrence: Return of cancer after its apparent disappearance.

Remission: Disappearance of detectable disease.

Sentinel node biopsy: Sentinel lymph node is removed and analyzed to determine if cancer has spread to other nodes.

Side effect: Unintentional or undesirable secondary effect of treatment.

Silicone: Synthetic material used in breast implants.

Stages of breast cancer: Used to describe the extent of the disease and if the cancer has spread, ranging from Stage 0 (mildest) to Stage IV (advanced).

Tattoo: Small, permanent dots on skin that outline the radiation treatment field.

TRAM flap (Trans rectus abdominous muscle): Reconstruction after mastectomy by transplanting abdominal flap to create a new breast.

Tumor: An abnormal growth of tissue which may be either benign or malignant.

Ultrasound: The use of sound waves to produce images of body tissues.

Bibliography

Web sites and books for surfing and reading

Reputable web sites for the latest medical information, useful products, and helpful support groups:

www.bcaction.org

www.breastcancer.com (Traditional Chinese Medicine: Qigong, acupressure, foods, lifestyle)

www.breastcancer.org

www.cancer.gov (National Cancer Institute)

www.cancer.org (American Cancer Society, 1-800-ACS-2345)

www.cbcf.org (Canadian Breast Cancer Foundation)

www.cbcn.ca (Canadian Breast Cancer Network, English/French)

www.cdc.gov/cancer (assistance and links to screening services to underserved women, free or low-cost mammograms and Pap test)

www.chemochicks.com

www.DrWeil.com

www.fertilehope.com

www.headcovers.com (hats, caps, wigs, etc.)

www.HealingWell.com

www.ibcsupport.org (Inflammatory Breast Cancer help and support)

www.lbbc.org (Living Beyond Breast Cancer)

www.MenAgainstBreastCancer.org

www.ncsc.ca (Breast Cancer Society of Canada)

www.NewYouBoutique.com (mastectomy breast forms and bras, breast enhancers, swimwear)

www.OneHealthPublishing.com (alternative & holistic)

www.SusanLoveMD.org

www.WebMD.com

www.y-me.org (National breast cancer organization, hotline)

www.youngsurvival.org (Young Survival Coalition)

Medical information is constantly updated. Get the latest editions. Borrow books at your hospital cancer center library. Check www.amazon.com (used copies often available for pennies) for more information on the following medical and inspirational titles recommended by survivors participating in this book:

Mitch Albom, *Tuesdays With Morrie:* An old man, a young man, and life's greatest lesson (Doubleday, 1997)

Greg Anderson, *Cancer:* 50 Essential Things to Do (Plume Books, 1999)

Melody Beattie, *The Language of Letting Go* (Hazelden Meditation Series, Hazelden, 1996)

Karen Berger, John Bostwick, *A Woman's Decision:* Breast care, treatment & reconstruction (St.Martin's Griffin, 1998)

Jean Shinoda Bolen, *Close to the Bone:* Life threatening illness and the search for meaning (Scribner, 1998)

Pema Chödrön; Eastern Philosophy Shambhala Classics, *The Places That Scare You:* A guide to fearlessness in difficult times (Shambhala, 2002); *Start Where You are:* A guide to compassionate living (Shambhala, 2001); *When Things Fall Apart:* Heart advice for difficult times (Shambala, 2000); *The Wisdom of No Escape:* And the path of loving kindness (Shambhala, 2001)

Deborah A. Cohen, Dr. Robert M. Geldfand, *Just Get Me Through This:* The practical guide to breast cancer (Kensington Publishing Corporation, 2001)

Sherry Lebed Davis, Stephanie Gunning, *Thriving After Breast Cancer:* Essential healing exercises for body and mind (Broadway, 2002)

Barbara Delinsky, *Uplift:* Secrets from the sisterhood of breast cancer survivor (Atria, 2001)

Viktor E. Frankl, *Man's Search for Meaning* (Pocket, 1997)

Vickie Girard, *There's No Place Like Hope:* A guide to beating cancer in mind-sized bites, A book of hope, help, and inspiration for cancer patients and their families (Compendium Publishing & Communications, 2001)

Thich Nhat Hahn, *Peace is Every Step:* The path of mindfulness in everyday life (Bantam, 1992)

Jimmie Holland and Sheldon Lewis, *The Human Side of Cancer:* Living with hope, coping with uncertainty (Perennial Currents, 2001)

Jon Kabat-Zinn, *Wherever You Go, There You Are:* Mindfulness meditation in everyday life (Hyperion, 1995)

Ronnie Kaye, *Spinning Straw Into Gold:* Your emotional recovery from breast cancer (Fireside, 1991)

Michael Lerner, *Choices in Healing:* Integrating the best of conventional and complementary approaches to cancer (The MIT Press, 1996)

Stephen Levine, *A Year to Live:* How to live this year as if it were your last (Harmony/Bell Tower, 1998)

John S. Link, et al, *Breast Cancer Survival Manual:* A step-by-step guide for the woman with newly diagnosed breast cancer (Owl Books, 2003)

Susan M. Love, et al, *Dr. Susan Love's Breast Book* (Harper Collins Publishers, 2000)

Nan Lu with Ellen Schaplowsky, *Traditional Chinese Medicine:* A woman's guide to healing from breast cancer (Avon Books, 1999)

Dawna Markova, *I Will Not Die an Unlived Life:* Reclaiming purpose and passion (Conari Press, 2000)

Beth Murphy, *Fighting for Our Future:* How young women find strength, hope, and courage while taking control of breast cancer (McGraw-Hill, 2003)

Joseph Murphy, *The Power of Your Subconscious Mind* (Bantam, 2001)

Caroline Myss, *Anatomy of the Spirit:* The seven stages of power and healing (Three Rivers Press, 1997)

Christiane Northrup, *Women's Bodies, Women's Wisdom* (Bantam, 1998)

M. Scott Peck, *The Road Less Traveled:* A new psychology of love, traditional values and spiritual growth (Touchstone, 2003)

Gilda Radner, *It's Always Something* (Simon & Schuster, 1989)

Rachel Naomi Remen, *Kitchen Table Wisdom:* Stories that heal (Riverhead Books, 1997); *My Grandfather's Blessings:* Stories of strength, refuge, and belonging (Riverhead Trade, 2001)

Martin L. Rossman, M.D., *Fighting Cancer From Within:* How to use the power of your mind for healing (Owl Books, 2003)

Hester Hill Licsw Schnipper, *After Breast Cancer:* A common-sense guide to life after treatment (Bantam, 2003)

Martin Seligman, *Learned Optimism:* How to change your mind and your life (Free Press, 1998)

Bernie S. Siegel, *Love, Medicine and Miracles:* Lessons learned about self-healing from a surgeon's experience with exceptional patients (Quill, 1990)

Philip Simmons, *Learning to Fall:* The blessings of an imperfect life (Bantam, 2003)

O. Carl Simonton, et al, *Getting Well Again:* The bestselling classic about the Simontons' revolutionary lifesaving self-awareness technique (Bantam, 1992)

Sharon Sorenson, Suzanne Metzger, *The Complete Idiot's Guide to Living with Breast Cancer* (Alpha Books, 2000)

Joan Swirsky, Diane Sackett Nannery, *Coping With Lymphedema* (Avery Publishing Group, 1998)

Mary Tagliaferri, Debu Tripathy, Isaac Cohen, *Breast Cancer Beyond Convention:* The world's foremost authorities on complementary and alternative medicine offer advice on healing (Atria, 2002)

Sue Patton Thoele, *The Courage to Be Yourself:* A woman's guide to emotional strength and self-esteem (Conari Press, 2001)

Eckhart Tolle, *The Power of Now:* A guide to spiritual enlightenment (New World Library, 2004)

Laura Jensen Walker, *Thanks for the Mammogram!* Fighting cancer with faith, hope, and a healthy dose of laughter (Revell, 2000)

Neale Donald Walsch, *Conversations with God:* An uncommon dialogue, Book 1 (Putnam Publishing Group, 1996), Book 2 (Hampton Roads Publishing Company 1997)

Dr. Andrew Weil, *Spontaneous Healing:* How to discover and embrace your body's natural ability to maintain and heal itself (Ballantine Books, 2000)

Marisa Weiss, Ellen Weiss, *Living Beyond Breast Cancer:* A survivor's guide for when treatment ends and the rest of your life begins (Three River Press, 1998)

Acknowledgments

I was not alone. I got much help through my cancer journey and in putting this book together. I am grateful for the support of my family and friends, and for the special contributions from the survivors.

First, of course, to my children, Albert and Rina Maarit Albala, who became my tireless supporters during the cancer crisis. They stood by me with infinite patience when the going got tough from the diagnosis to the treatments and beyond, and they pulled me back to life again. They always knew intuitively what to say and what to do. And to their partners, Lydie Servanin and James Awad. All four have helped in many practical and emotional ways with this book, to prepare the questionnaire and get it online for electronic responses, with much needed enthusiastic feedback and help about ongoing progress.

My husband, Elie, even though we are separated, was there for me and helped me in many practical ways with loving kindness. It gave me strength to know I could count on him, and it was important for our children, too. We all got through the crisis as a strong, united family.

To my three sisters in Finland, Maarit, Anita, and Arja. All of them gave me incredible support throughout my journey, through emails and phone calls, including an uplifting visit from Maarit during my treatments, to remind me that I am an important part of their lives. To my niece, Saila Reiniö, for visiting me in the aftermath and for listening to my childhood stories, bringing the past back to life for me— remembering the past is important since it makes the cancer crisis what it is, just temporary. To Kerttu and Bill Thorne, my cousin and her husband, who called often and sent many loving letters and delightful cards during my treatments to make me laugh and to remind me that they too were rooting for me.

To my caring friends near and far, Kay Turner, Donna Tremblay, Doris Aschenbach, Margareta Tallberg, Michelle West, Sheila Mullin, Maddy Cranley, Helen Gauthier, Angelica Fovero, Margaret Treder, Juliet Gauthier, Ulla Lehtonen, Mia Katariina Linden, Christina Manolescu, and Julie Northey.

For excellent suggestions and professional feedback on the questionnaire and final draft, to Bev Parker. Bev also wrote the foreword for this book, perfectly capturing the essence of my work and conveying the message of this book to others. Also to Shelagh Coinner, Kay Turner, Donna Tremblay, Michelle West, and MaryAnn Browne. Your comments, proofreading, and feedback helped me to make the questionnaire and the book user-friendly and relevant, focusing on what matters.

To my many doctors, nurses, and technicians at the hospital for taking such good care of me. I now have a new understanding and appreciation of your often difficult work and long hours with gravely ill people in distress all needing your time, help, experience, and attention. To Lymphedema Association of Quebec for information on lymphedema. And to my remarkable pharmacist, Christine, for taking personal interest in me and my health, and for calmly giving me truthful information when I got tired and confused.

To all those who loved my project from the start and spread the word about this book to bring responses to me. I will never even know who you all are, but I am grateful for your invisible and invaluable network which helped make this project such a success.

And, most importantly, to 125 women who responded to my invitation and participated in this book—and also to two men who had lost their wives to breast cancer and responded briefly and unexpectedly. I received more than 2,000 pages of stories, tips, and glimpses from your cancer journeys to make this book what it is, interesting and honest. I was only able to use a portion of each response to keep this book manageable in size and yet give voice to everyone. Thank you for your time and caring. Whether you have used your full name, first name, initials, pseudonym, or chose to be anonymous—the options I offered to protect the privacy of participants, every comment is appreciated with profound gratitude. You have made this book possible and a voice of many to help others. May you live long and healthy lives.

Index

Aftermath 136
Aftermath tips:
Allowing yourself
to mourn 137
BSE 138
Embracing
life 137
Exercising 138
Facing stress 137
Itchy, dry skin 138
Journaling 137
Laughter and
tears 138
Muscle stiffness,
aches, pains 139
Music and art 138
Professional
help 139
Reduce stress 139
Relax cautiously
139
Taking a break 137
Talking 138
Water therapy 139
Afterthoughts 207
Appointments 33
Bibliography 216
Brief profiles 12
**First reactions,
survivor tips** 12
Chemotherapy 76
Chemotherapy tips:

Aversion to
food 78
Bald head 82
Body odor 83
Comfort tips 82
Constipation and
diarrhea 81
Dry mouth 80
Emotional help 85
Exercise 84
Food & drinks 79
Getting help 84
Hair loss 82
Hydration 78
Infections 78
Mouth sores 80
Nausea 81
Pains, aches 81
Port-a-cath 78
Rest, work 83
Side effects 77
Sleep 83
Stress relief 84
Support for
sessions 85
Taking time out 84
Tooth care 80
Visits 85
Vitamins 77
Warning signs 77
Clinical trials 33
Complementary and

**alternative
treatments** 107
**Dealing with the
medical system** 33
**Diagnosis, events
surrounding** 12
Facing death 190
Fear of recurrence
116
Survivor tips 117
Glossary 214
**Heatbag,
microwavable** 91
**Hormonal therapy
drugs** 99
Humor 198
Introduction 10
**Life-changing
moment** 12
Lumpectomy 47
Lymphedema 69
Lymphedema tips:
Activities 71
Avoiding it 71
Danger signs 72
Exercises 71
Prognosis and
treatment 72
Protect yourself 70
Sun and insects 70
Swelling 72
Who is at risk 70

Mastectomy 53
Moving away from
illness 171
Optimism and
pessimism 127
Survivor tips 128
Patient (what makes
a good patient) 34
Radiation 92
Radiation tips:
Avoid 93
Backache during
sessions 96
Bathing 96
Care after 96
Clothing 98
Cooling radiated
area 95
Creams 94
Dehydration 97
Dry mouth 97
Fatigue 94
Inconvenience 93
Ink markings 93
Nausea 97
Perfumes 97
Perspiration 96
Posttreatment 97
Shaving 95
Sleep 93
Sun exposure 95
Tattooing 93
Tips from nurse 92

Reclaiming life 171
Survivor tips 172
Joys today 174
Reconstruction
53, 55
Recurrence,
fear 116
Regaining arm
movement 66
Exercise tips 50
Spirituality 185
Support 149
Support tips:
Best gifts 155
Best things
to say 157
What can help 153
Who can help 149
Worst things
to say 160
Surgeries 46
Surgery tips:
Bathing and
bandages 54
Bra tips and breast
enhancers 47-48
Clothing 47
Cold breast 49
Drains 47, 50
Frozen shoulder
50
Going home 49
Exercises to regain

arm movement 51
Help after
major surgery 54
Massage 55
Numbness 52
Nutrition 55
Pain after
surgery 52
Pampering 54
Patience after
treatments 53
Pictures of being
bald 54
Prostheses and
other options 48
Reconstruction 55
Regaining arm
movement 50, 66
Resting after 49
Scar care 53
Tingly, itchy, numb
underarm 53
What helps 55
Tamoxifen and
aromatase
inhibitors 99
Survivor tips 99
Hot flashes 100
Leg cramps 101
Vaginal dryness,
itching 101
Using this book 5
Web sites 216

Please visit www.dancingwithfear.org

- for individual and quantity orders
- for feedback about this book
- to participate in *Dancing With Fear: Tips and wisdom from breast cancer survivors, Volume II*
- to participate in *Dancing With Fear: Tips and wisdom from families and friends of breast cancer survivors*